# Integrating Systems and Sectors Toward Obesity Solutions

## PROCEEDINGS OF A WORKSHOP

Emily A. Callahan, *Rapporteur*

Roundtable on Obesity Solutions

Food and Nutrition Board

Health and Medicine Division

*The National Academies of*
SCIENCES · ENGINEERING · MEDICINE

THE NATIONAL ACADEMIES PRESS
*Washington, DC*
**www.nap.edu**

THE NATIONAL ACADEMIES PRESS    500 Fifth Street, NW    Washington, DC 20001

This activity was partially supported by the Academy of Nutrition and Dietetics; Alliance for a Healthier Generation; American Academy of Pediatrics; American College of Sports Medicine; American Council on Exercise; American Society for Nutrition; Banner Health; Bipartisan Policy Center; BlueCross BlueShield of North Carolina Foundation; Blue Shield of California Foundation; The California Endowment; General Mills, Inc.; Greater Rochester Health Foundation; Intermountain Healthcare; The JPB Foundation; The Kresge Foundation; Mars, Inc.; National Recreation and Park Association; Nemours; Novo Nordisk; Obesity Action Coalition; The Obesity Society; Partnership for a Healthier America; Reinvestment Fund; Robert Wood Johnson Foundation; SHAPE America; Society of Behavioral Medicine; Wake Forest Baptist Medical Center; Walmart; WW International, Inc.; and YMCA of the USA. Any opinions, findings, conclusions, or recommendations expressed in this publication do not necessarily reflect the views of any organization or agency that provided support for the project.

International Standard Book Number-13: 978-0-309-67620-5
International Standard Book Number-10: 0-309-67620-7
Digital Object Identifier: https://doi.org/10.17226/25766

Additional copies of this publication are available from the National Academies Press, 500 Fifth Street, NW, Keck 360, Washington, DC 20001; (800) 624-6242 or (202) 334-3313; http://www.nap.edu.

Suggested citation: National Academies of Sciences, Engineering, and Medicine. 2021. *Integrating systems and sectors toward obesity solutions: Proceedings of a workshop.* Washington, DC: The National Academies Press. https://doi.org/10.17226/25766.

*The National Academies of*
# SCIENCES · ENGINEERING · MEDICINE

The **National Academy of Sciences** was established in 1863 by an Act of Congress, signed by President Lincoln, as a private, nongovernmental institution to advise the nation on issues related to science and technology. Members are elected by their peers for outstanding contributions to research. Dr. Marcia McNutt is president.

The **National Academy of Engineering** was established in 1964 under the charter of the National Academy of Sciences to bring the practices of engineering to advising the nation. Members are elected by their peers for extraordinary contributions to engineering. Dr. John L. Anderson is president.

The **National Academy of Medicine** (formerly the Institute of Medicine) was established in 1970 under the charter of the National Academy of Sciences to advise the nation on medical and health issues. Members are elected by their peers for distinguished contributions to medicine and health. Dr. Victor J. Dzau is president.

The three Academies work together as the **National Academies of Sciences, Engineering, and Medicine** to provide independent, objective analysis and advice to the nation and conduct other activities to solve complex problems and inform public policy decisions. The National Academies also encourage education and research, recognize outstanding contributions to knowledge, and increase public understanding in matters of science, engineering, and medicine.

Learn more about the National Academies of Sciences, Engineering, and Medicine at **www.nationalacademies.org**.

*The National Academies of*
## SCIENCES · ENGINEERING · MEDICINE

**Consensus Study Reports** published by the National Academies of Sciences, Engineering, and Medicine document the evidence-based consensus on the study's statement of task by an authoring committee of experts. Reports typically include findings, conclusions, and recommendations based on information gathered by the committee and the committee's deliberations. Each report has been subjected to a rigorous and independent peer-review process and it represents the position of the National Academies on the statement of task.

**Proceedings** published by the National Academies of Sciences, Engineering, and Medicine chronicle the presentations and discussions at a workshop, symposium, or other event convened by the National Academies. The statements and opinions contained in proceedings are those of the participants and are not endorsed by other participants, the planning committee, or the National Academies.

For information about other products and activities of the National Academies, please visit www.nationalacademies.org/about/whatwedo.

# PLANNING COMMITTEE ON INTEGRATING SYSTEMS AND SECTORS TOWARD OBESITY SOLUTIONS[1]

**CHRISTINA ECONOMOS** (*Co-Chair*), Co-Founder and Director, ChildObesity180 and Professor and New Balance Chair in Childhood Nutrition, Friedman School of Nutrition Science and Policy, Tufts University

**NICOLAAS (NICO) PRONK** (*Co-Chair*), President, HealthPartners Institute and Chief Science Officer, HealthPartners

**SARA BLEICH,** Professor of Public Health Policy, Harvard T.H. Chan School of Public Health and Carol K. Pforzheimer Professor, Radcliffe Institute for Advanced Study

**GISELLE CORBIE-SMITH,** Kenan Distinguished Professor of Social Medicine, Director of Center for Health Equity Research, and Professor of Internal Medicine, University of North Carolina at Chapel Hill

**SARA CZAJA,** Professor of Gerontology in Medicine and Director of the Center on Aging and Behavioral Research, Weill Cornell Medical College

**APRIL OH,** Senior Advisor for Implementation Science and Health Equity, Division of Cancer Control and Population Sciences, National Cancer Institute, National Institutes of Health

**DANIEL E. RIVERA,** Professor of Chemical Engineering and Program Director of the Control Systems Engineering Laboratory, Arizona State University

*Health and Medicine Division Staff*

**LESLIE J. SIM,** Roundtable Director (*through December 2020*)
**HEATHER DEL VALLE COOK,** Roundtable Director
**AMANDA NGUYEN,** Program Officer
**MEREDITH YOUNG,** Research Associate
**CYPRESS LYNX,** Research Associate
**ZARIA FYFFE,** Senior Program Assistant

---

[1]The National Academies of Sciences, Engineering, and Medicine's planning committees are solely responsible for organizing the workshop, identifying topics, and choosing speakers. The responsibility for the published Proceedings of a Workshop rests with the workshop rapporteur and the institution.

# ROUNDTABLE ON OBESITY SOLUTIONS[1]

**NICOLAAS (NICO) PRONK** (*Chair*), HealthPartners Institute and HealthPartners, Bloomington, Minnesota

**CHRISTINA ECONOMOS** (*Vice Chair*), Tufts University, Boston, Massachusetts

**IHUOMA ENELI** (*Vice Chair*), American Academy of Pediatrics, Columbus, Ohio

**SHARON ADAMS-TAYLOR,** The School Superintendents Association, Alexandria, Virginia

**KATIE ADAMSON,** YMCA of the USA, Washington, DC

**JAMY D. ARD,** Wake Forest University, Winston-Salem, North Carolina

**DANIELLE BERMAN,** Food and Nutrition Service, U.S. Food and Drug Administration, Washington, DC

**ROBIN P. BLACKSTONE,** University of Arizona, Phoenix, Arizona

**HEIDI MICHELS BLANCK,** Centers for Disease Control and Prevention, Atlanta, Georgia

**JEANNE BLANKENSHIP,** Academy of Nutrition and Dietetics, Washington, DC

**SARA N. BLEICH,** Harvard T.H. Chan School of Public Health, Boston, Massachusetts

**DON W. BRADLEY,** Duke University, Durham, North Carolina

**HEIDI F. BURKE,** Greater Rochester Health Foundation, Rochester, New York

**JAMIE BUSSEL,** Robert Wood Johnson Foundation, Princeton, New Jersey

**MERRY DAVIS,** BlueCross BlueShield of North Carolina Foundation, Durham, North Carolina

**JENNIFER FASSBENDER,** Reinvestment Fund, Philadelphia, Pennsylvania

**AMENDA FISHER,** Walmart, Betonville, Arkansas

**GARY D. FOSTER,** WW International, Inc., New York, New York

**DAVID D. FUKUZAWA,** The Kresge Foundation, Troy, Michigan

**ALLISON GERTEL-ROSENBERG,** Nemours Children's Health System, Washington, DC

**MARJORIE A. INNOCENT,** National Association for the Advancement of Colored People, Baltimore, Maryland

**JOHN JAKICIC,** University of Pittsburgh, Pennsylvania

**ELIZABETH A. JOY,** Intermountain Healthcare, Salt Lake City, Utah

**SCOTT I. KAHAN,** The George Washington University, Washington, DC

---

[1] The National Academies of Sciences, Engineering, and Medicine's forums and roundtables do not issue, review, or approve individual documents. The responsibility for the published Proceedings of a Workshop rests with the workshop rapporteur and the institution.

PETER T. KATZMARZYK, Pennington Biomedical Research Center, Baton Rouge, Louisiana
CATHERINE KWIK-URIBE, Mars, Inc., Germantown, Maryland
THEODORE KYLE, The Obesity Society, Pittsburgh, Pennsylvania
LISEL LOY, Bipartisan Policy Center, Washington, DC
KELLIE MAY, National Recreation and Park Association, Ashburn, Virginia
MYETA M. MOON, United Way Worldwide, Alexandria, Virginia
STEPHANIE A. MORRIS, SHAPE America, Reston, Virginia
JOSEPH NADGLOWSKI, JR., Obesity Action Coalition, Tampa, Florida
MELISSA NAPOLITANO, The George Washington University, Washington, DC
PATRICIA NECE, Obesity Action Coalition, Tampa, Florida
MEGAN NECHANICKY, General Mills, Inc., Minneapolis, Minnesota
BARBARA PICOWER, The JPB Foundation, New York, New York
SUE P. POLIS, National League of Cities, Washington, DC
AMELIE G. RAMIREZ, Salud America!, San Antonio, Texas
TOM RICHARDS, American Council on Exercise, San Diego, California
NANCY ROMAN, Partnership for a Healthier America, Washington, DC
SYLVIA ROWE, SR Strategy, LLC, Washington, DC
LAURIE STRADLEY, Alliance for a Healthier Generation, Asheville, North Carolina
SUSAN Z. YANOVSKI, National Institute of Diabetes and Digestive and Kidney Diseases, National Institutes of Health, Bethesda, Maryland
LESLIE ZOLOV, Novo Nordisk, Washington, DC

*Health and Medicine Division Staff*

LESLIE J. SIM, Roundtable Director (*through December 2020*)
HEATHER DEL VALLE COOK, Roundtable Director
AMANDA NGUYEN, Program Officer
MEREDITH YOUNG, Research Associate
CYPRESS LYNX, Research Associate
ZARIA FYFFE, Senior Program Assistant
ANN L. YAKTINE, Director, Food and Nutrition Board

*Food and Nutrition Board Liaison*

SHIRIKI KUMANYIKA, Drexel University, Philadelphia, Pennsylvania

*Consultant*

WILLIAM (BILL) H. DIETZ, The George Washington University, Washington, DC

# Reviewers

This Proceedings of a Workshop was reviewed in draft form by individuals chosen for their diverse perspectives and technical expertise. The purpose of this independent review is to provide candid and critical comments that will assist the National Academies of Sciences, Engineering, and Medicine in making each published proceedings as sound as possible and to ensure that it meets the institutional standards for quality, objectivity, evidence, and responsiveness to the charge. The review comments and draft manuscript remain confidential to protect the integrity of the process.

We thank the following individuals for their review of this proceedings:

**LARISSA CALANCIE,** Tufts University
**PATTY MABRY,** HealthPartners Institute
**JODI MITCHELL,** JC Health Strategies

Although the reviewers listed above provided many constructive comments and suggestions, they were not asked to endorse the content of the proceedings, nor did they see the final draft before its release. The review of this proceedings was overseen by **SHARI BARKIN,** Vanderbilt University Medical Center. She was responsible for making certain that an independent examination of this proceedings was carried out in accordance with standards of the National Academies and that all review comments were carefully considered. Responsibility for the final content rests entirely with the rapporteur and the National Academies.

# Contents

# Boxes and Figures

# 1

# Introduction

A virtual workshop titled Integrating Systems and Sectors Toward Obesity Solutions, held April 6, 2020 (Part I), and June 30, 2020 (Part II), was convened by the Roundtable on Obesity Solutions, Health and Medicine Division, National Academies of Sciences, Engineering, and Medicine. The workshop introduced the concept of complex systems and the field of systems science, and explored systems science approaches to obesity solutions. Speakers provided an overview of systems science theories, approaches, and applications, highlighting examples from within and outside the obesity field. Presentations and discussions examined complex systems in society that have the potential to shape public health and well-being, and considered opportunities for systems change as they relate to obesity solutions. Specifically, the workshop explored factors that can influence obesity—such as (in)equity, relationships, connections, networks, capacity, power dynamics, social determinants, and political will—and how these factors can impact communications and cross-sector collaboration to address obesity. The workshop's Statement of Task is in Box 1-1.[1]

---

[1]The workshop agenda, presentations, and other materials are available at https://www.nationalacademies.org/event/04-06-2020/integrating-systems-and-sectors-toward-obesity-solutions-part-1 (accessed October 5, 2020) and https://www.nationalacademies.org/event/06-30-2020/integrating-systems-and-sectors-toward-obesity-solutions-part-2 (accessed October 5, 2020).

---

**BOX 1-1**
**Workshop Statement of Task**

A planning committee of the National Academies of Sciences, Engineering, and Medicine will plan and conduct a 1-day public workshop that will feature invited presentations and discussions to (1) introduce the concept of complex systems science and (2) consider systems science approaches to obesity solutions.

Workshop presentations will provide a background on systems science theories and applications and will feature examples from within and outside of the obesity field. Presentations and discussions will explore complex systems in society that have the potential to shape the health and well-being of the population and will consider opportunities for change as they relate to obesity solutions. The workshop will explore complex systems and contributing factors that can influence obesity (including the roles played by (in)equity, relationships, connections, networks, capacity, power dynamics, social determinants, and political will) and their impact on effective communications and cross-sector collaboration.

---

## INTRODUCTORY REMARKS

Nicolaas (Nico) Pronk, president of HealthPartners Institute, chief science officer at HealthPartners, and chair of the Roundtable on Obesity Solutions, welcomed workshop participants and provided a brief overview of the roundtable, explaining that it engages leaders and voices from diverse sectors (e.g., health care, health insurance, academia, business, education, child care, government, media, philanthropy, nonprofit) to help solve the nation's obesity crisis. Through meetings, public workshops, reports, and four innovation collaboratives,[2] he continued, the roundtable provides a venue for ongoing dialogue on critical and emerging issues in obesity prevention, as well as treatment and weight maintenance.

Pronk noted that since the roundtable commenced in 2014, its discussions and publications have covered a number of topics including the scientific basis for obesity, research gaps, the current state of obesity solutions, and ways to drive further progress and overcome challenges in implementation and scalability. In particular, the roundtable has highlighted promising multisector policy, systems, and environmental approaches, with a focus on sustainable, equitable strategies for addressing obesity-related disparities.

---

[2]Innovation collaboratives engage participants with similar interests and responsibilities in cooperative activities to advance aspects of a roundtable's Statement of Task. These ad hoc convening activities foster information sharing and collaboration toward the roundtable's aims.

In 2019, Pronk continued, the roundtable explored broader cross-cutting issues, including communication strategies and health equity approaches. These issues, he said, led the roundtable to adopt and apply a multisector systems perspective on ways to advance, diffuse, and sustain effective obesity solutions. He explained that the roundtable's 2020 plans include developing a systems map and holding a follow-on workshop addressing how systems modeling approaches can inform obesity research and solutions. These activities will culminate in a strategic roadmap to action in which various stakeholders can identify places to act, intervene, and coordinate with others in the system.

## ORGANIZATION OF THIS PROCEEDINGS

This proceedings follows the order of the workshop agendas (see Appendix A), chronicling its sessions in individual chapters. Chapter 2 presents an overview of systems science theories, approaches, and applications. Chapter 3 explores complex systems in society and contributing factors that can influence obesity, including power dynamics, structural racism, relationships (e.g., interpersonal, familial, community, professional), resources, place-based issues, policy, and political will. Chapter 4 examines how complex systems may influence obesity and considers opportunities for systems change as they relate to obesity solutions. Finally, Chapter 5 highlights research activities that apply systems thinking to address obesity and population health and well-being. In addition to Appendix A, three other appendixes are included. Appendix B is a list of acronyms and abbreviations used in this proceedings; Appendix C includes a glossary and a bibliography of background resources related to systems science theories, approaches, and applications; and Appendix D provides the biographical sketches of the workshop speakers and the planning committee members.

# 2

# Overview of Systems Science Theories, Approaches, and Applications

---

**Highlights from the Presentations of Individual Speakers**

- The complex nature of many public health problems, including obesity, makes them well suited to examination with systems science approaches. Such approaches can help in tackling the challenges of coordinating policy and action across sectors, cultivating interdisciplinary connections, and navigating heterogeneity across settings. Systems science approaches in the context of obesity can help inform the sustainable, effective implementation of tailored, adaptive multifaceted and whole-of-community interventions. (Ross Hammond)
- Multiple forces drive population health epidemics such as obesity. Therefore, the use of complex lenses to identify systemic insights and key levers for intervention will achieve maximal impact to improve population health and narrow health inequities. Systems science approaches can complement observational and experimental techniques to simulate the counterfactual scenarios in which one variable is changed while all others are held constant, thereby advancing understanding of strategies for improving population health. (Sandro Galea)
- Using systems thinking and approaches to study chronic disease enhances exploration of the role of context, facilitates examination of underlying causal mechanisms, and produces tools with high relevance for community stakeholders and

---

policy makers. Understanding causal mechanisms can lead to more effective intervention and policy design, support advocacy efforts toward maintaining or terminating programs, and illuminate the processes through which health disparities arise. (Douglas Luke)

Part I of the workshop was an introductory session, moderated by Daniel E. Rivera, professor of chemical engineering and program director of the Control Systems Engineering Laboratory at Arizona State University. Speakers in this session introduced the concepts of complex systems and systems thinking as they apply to population health issues and broadly described systems science approaches (i.e., methodologies or tools) that could be applied to obesity solutions. (These key terms, defined in Box 2-1, were used throughout the workshop. See Appendix D for a full glossary of terms used by workshop speakers.) Three speakers delivered presentations, engaged in a panel discussion, and answered questions from workshop participants.

## OVERVIEW AND HISTORY OF SYSTEMS SCIENCE

Ross Hammond, the Betty Bofinger Brown Associate Professor at Washington University in St. Louis and director of the Center on Social Dynamics and Policy and senior fellow in economics at the Brookings

---

**BOX 2-1**
**Key Terms Used in the Workshop**
*Presented by Christina Economos, Tufts University*

**Complex systems** are comprised of heterogeneous elements that interact with each other. Those interactions produce an effect that is distinct from the effects of the individual elements.

**Systems science approaches** are a broad class of analytical approaches (i.e., methodologies or tools) that aim to uncover the behavior of complex systems. A distinction is made between *hard* systems methods, such as quantitative dynamic model building, and *soft* systems methods, such as qualitative, action-based research methods.

**Systems thinking** is a broad paradigm concerned with interrelationships, perspectives, and boundaries. It recognizes that a system has interrelated, interdependent parts that can function synergistically.

Institution, presented a historical overview of systems science, including its advantages and potential applications to public health and obesity research and intervention. The multifaceted nature of many public health problems—including the obesity epidemic—makes them challenging for scientists and policy makers to address, he stated, adding that such intricate complexity makes these problems well suited to examination with systems science approaches.

Hammond described four characteristics of complex systems such as those that drive obesity. First, he began, many different factors interact across multiple sectors and scales to affect relevant behaviors and outcomes, the result of which is a deeply interconnected system. As an example, he showed a diagram constructed by the United Kingdom. Foresight Group to map measurable factors that drive obesity (see Figure 2-1). He pointed out the interconnected and interdependent system illustrated by this map, noting that an isolated focus on a single part of such a system risks missing many other important factors and linkages.

The second characteristic, Hammond continued, is that complex systems include multiple heterogeneous actors who may affect obesity outcomes, such as individual consumers, retailers, schools, health care providers, and community coalition leaders. These actors have different incentives, information, and network connections, he observed, explaining that their interconnections are important because an intervention may unintentionally affect certain actors, with implications for their connections with other actors. Actors are also adaptive, Hammond added, elaborating that differences may exist between their short- and long-term behavioral responses to environmental and policy changes.

Hammond described a third characteristic of complex systems by stressing the importance of detailed information with regard to the context and timing of various exposures as people move through their environments. To illustrate this point, he showed a map of average exposure to fast food outlets across five boroughs of New York City, pointing out the richness of information it reflected. If the map were collapsed into zip code averages for density of fast food outlets, he said, it would conceal important details about how people move through a space and experience its food environment. The structure of people's lived experiences matters, he underscored, noting that social networks are another example of a structure that affects the development of obesity.

Lastly, Hammond highlighted the dynamic nature of complex systems. He stressed the potential importance of the timing and sequence of exposures and interventions as related to the development of obesity and other chronic disease outcomes across the lifespan.

Turning to the implications of applying systems science approaches to obesity, Hammond emphasized that searching for a single cause of a

8

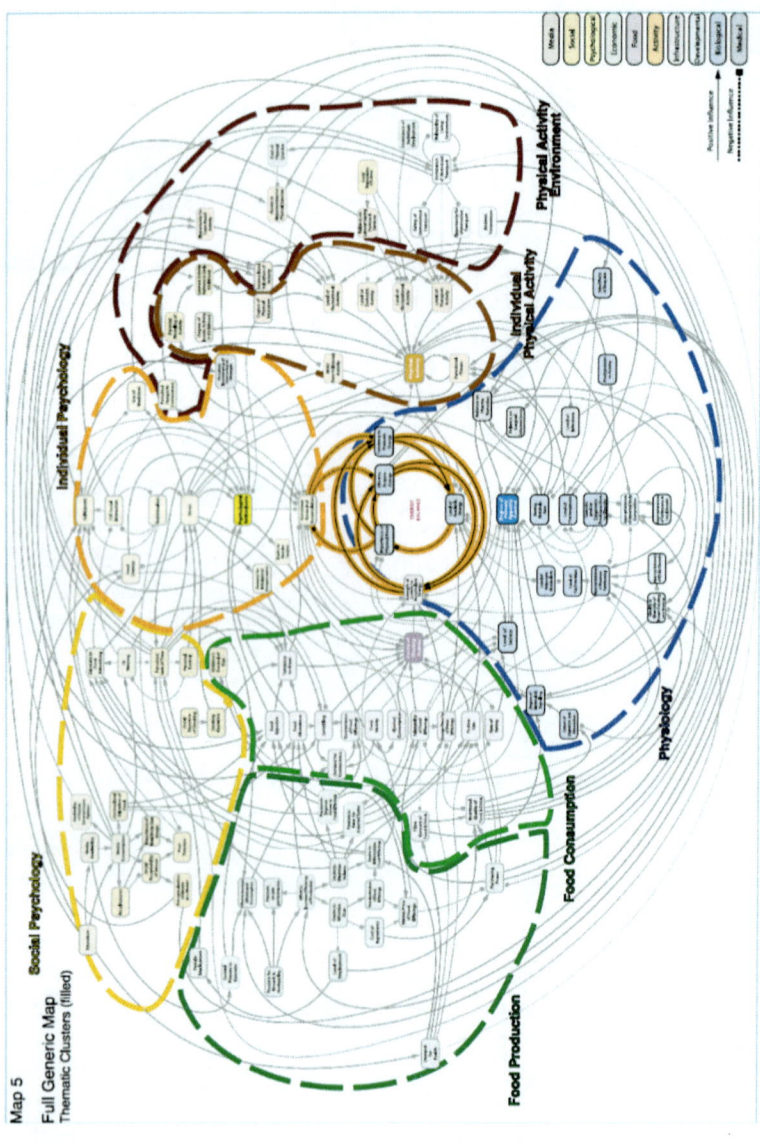

**FIGURE 2-1** Map of measurable factors that drive obesity.
SOURCES: Presented by Ross Hammond, April 6, 2020. United Kingdom Government Office for Science, 2007.
<http://www.foresight.gov.uk/OurWork/ActiveProjects/Obesity/KeyInfo/Index.asp>

problem driven by a complex system is often misleading. Furthermore, he added, standard tools focused on single drivers may have limited ability to capture obesity's complexity. Thus, he said, a growing consensus supports solutions that are broad enough to address a variety of contributing factors while also being sufficiently tailored to specific contexts and adaptive over time.

To support these points, Hammond referenced a series of reports endorsing the use of complex systems thinking, approaches, and models to inform solutions for obesity and other public health issues. These include several publications of the Institute of Medicine and the National Academies, particularly a 2012 report titled *Accelerating Progress in Obesity Prevention* (IOM, 2012) and a report on the use of systems science approaches in tobacco regulation (IOM, 2015), as well as a Healthy People 2030 report from the Department of Health and Human Services (Secretary's Advisory Committee for Healthy People 2030, 2018) (see also IOM, 2012, 2015; IOM and NRC, 2015; NASEM, 2016; United Kingdom Government Office for Science, 2007). Hammond also mentioned that the National Institutes of Health (NIH) has invested in at least five networks of scientists who have applied systems science approaches to various issues.

Hammond proposed that the interest in systems science approaches is driven by a desire to support the selection of policies and solutions that leverage or at least address the complexity of the problems they seek to address. He elaborated that these approaches can help tackle the challenges of coordinating policy and action across sectors, cultivating connections among scientific disciplines, and navigating heterogeneity across settings.

Hammond drew a distinction between the terms "systems science" and "systems thinking" as applied to public health. He described the latter term as an approach to thinking about the world as opposed to the use of quantitative or qualitative methods. Stakeholders applying systems thinking, he elaborated, examine complex systems from a holistic perspective and search for points of leverage and coordinated solutions beyond traditional arenas of health. Public health has advanced from using systems thinking, he explained, to adopting specific systems science tools, both qualitative and quantitative.

Hammond briefly mentioned causal loop diagrams and systems maps as examples of qualitative tools, and then reviewed quantitative tools in more detail. He highlighted the existence of a great diversity of quantitative tools and implementation methodologies, referencing a listing of some of these methods, along with their potential uses, in the *Accelerating Progress in Obesity Prevention* report (IOM, 2012). All of these tools, he explained, embrace complexity and seek to understand the mechanisms that drive outcomes, but they differ in several respects. One difference is the perspective from which they seek to understand processes and outcomes, which he said may be from the top down, marked by interest in the system's structure, or from the bottom up, marked by interest in individual actors in that system and the fine details of how they interact. He identified as another difference the formalisms used, which include differential equations, a focus on network ties, and portrayals of individuals referred to as agents. Tools also differ in the relative emphasis they place on data inputs versus theoretical inputs, Hammond added, as well as their field of origin and the training required to use them. He noted that NIH's initial investment and training in systems science approaches focused on system dynamics modeling, social network models, and agent-based modeling, which remain among the most common types of methods used in public health and obesity.

Hammond briefly recapped the history of complex systems science, pointing out that many of its methods date back to the 1950s or earlier (with the exception, for example, of agent-based modeling, which originated in the 1990s). These methods emerged from such fields as biology, social science, and engineering, he said, where many of them established strong track records as policy- or decision-making support tools undergirded by empirical experiments across a wide variety of topics. He added that a catalyst in merging these fields and methods was the creation of the independent, nonprofit Santa Fe Institute in the 1980s, which is dedicated to the multidisciplinary study of fundamental principles of complex adaptive systems.

Systems science approaches were first used in public health to inform control and management of infectious diseases, Hammond observed, activity that accelerated after the September 11, 2001, terrorist attacks amid concerns about bioterrorism and pandemics. Further traction was gained with an investment by NIH that resulted in the creation of the MIDAS (Models of Infectious Disease Agent Study) network in 2003, which Hammond said has had important scientific and policy impacts. MIDAS makes extensive use of agent-based computational modeling, he noted, a systems science method that plays a key role in informing policy options related to the coronavirus disease 2019 (COVID-19) pandemic.

The models used by MIDAS were first summoned to inform policy solutions during the H1N1 crisis in 2009 and 2010, Hammond recounted, by which time they had undergone several years of development and improvement since the launch of MIDAS. He explained that this chronology suggests the time horizon for which these models might be expected to yield actionable results in the context of obesity solutions.

According to Hammond, systems science approaches have been applied to public health issues for three key purposes, which he said could guide thinking about the application of these approaches to obesity issues. One purpose is etiological, which, he explained, includes generating hypotheses and building theories to help uncover potentially unobservable mechanisms that drive behaviors or outcomes in the real world, informing future intervention targets, timing, dosage, and data collection needs and methods. The second purpose, Hammond continued, is to deduce retrospectively the key influences on an intervention's outcomes so as to better understand why it failed or succeeded, and to inform future data collection needs for evaluation and intervention design. Models used for this purpose, he added, can also inform the replication of successful intervention elements in different settings or over longer time horizons. A third purpose is prospective modeling, which Hammond described as helping to forecast potential outcomes of different policy and intervention options. He suggested that prospective modeling is a particularly attractive method for informing obesity solutions because it turns implicit mental models into explicit scenarios that harness a problem's complexity and help account for heterogeneity across individuals and settings. Furthermore, he continued, this virtual modeling may be more efficient, ethical, and/or cost-effective than conducting large-scale, real-world experiments.

Hammond shifted his exposition of systems science history to describe how obesity research has been informed by systems science approaches. Publications first appeared in this area around 2009, he remarked, and these initial publications explained why systems science approaches are apt for studying obesity and designing interventions to address it, reviewed potential applications of specific systems science methods and tools to obesity, and suggested potential data requirements and obstacles (Hammond, 2009). Within a short time, he said, an editorial in a special issue of the *American Journal of Public Health* (AJPH) argued that systems science approaches were a revolution for public health policy research (Mabry et al., 2010). Next, NIH funded a network of researchers who were using systems science approaches to examine the etiology of obesity; the results of this investment were reported in another special issue of AJPH in 2014 (Mabry and Bures, 2014). The policy implications of some of these models were reported in an obesity-focused issue of *The Lancet*, Hammond added, and the NIH-funded work on etiology has continued for obesity and other topics.

Hammond reported that the concept of complex systems modeling for obesity solutions entered mainstream consciousness in 2012 with the publication of the *Accelerating Progress in Obesity Prevention* report (IOM, 2012). He mentioned specific applications of this concept, including COMPACT (Childhood Obesity Modeling for Prevention and Community Transformation) (see Chapter 4); a paper advocating for combining systems science approaches that have complementary strengths (Hennessy et al., 2020); and two reviews describing current uses of complex systems modeling for efforts addressing obesity, diet, and food systems (Langellier et al., 2019; Morshed et al., 2019).

Years of investment, training, and collaboration have contributed to the evolution of systems science approaches in the context of obesity, Hammond maintained, noting that in the future, these approaches can inform the sustainable, effective implementation of multifaceted or whole-of-community interventions. Moreover, he argued, these approaches can enable disease prevention efforts that are as precise and tailored as disease treatments informed by precision medicine (Gillman and Hammond, 2016). Hammond concluded his presentation with the following quote:

> Furthermore, there is a need to train scientists in academia, the private sector, and government agencies in all aspects of complex systems approaches—including systems research design, data collection, and analytical methodologies—and the use of models appealing for private sector actors and government agencies to leverage systems science approaches. (IOM and NRC, 2015)

## SYSTEMS THINKING TO UNDERSTAND AND IMPROVE POPULATION HEALTH

Sandro Galea, dean and the Robert A. Knox Professor at the Boston University School of Public Health, discussed using systems thinking and systems science approaches to understand and improve population health. A fundamental point, he asserted, is that population health and its complex challenges, such as obesity, cannot be broadly understood without taking a systems science approach.

Galea asserted that systems science approaches are well suited to application to population health, which has been defined as "the health outcomes of a group of individuals, including the distribution of such outcomes within the group" (Kindig and Stoddart, 2003). Such approaches offer unique insights into the overall health of populations and the health inequities that exist within them, he elaborated, adding that these systemic insights are critical for informing interventions to improve public health.

Galea shared an illustration that he said represents typical, deterministic approaches to population health. He explained that such approaches do not apply complex systems lenses, and assume that all individuals are relatively interchangeable and lack specific network structures and interconnectivity. Furthermore, he added, these approaches are broadly predicated on an assumption of a linear relationship between exposure and outcome functions.

In reality, Galea pointed out, substituting one person for another could have vastly different effects in a given situation because populations are heterogeneous. They comprise markedly diverse individuals who have complex contact structures, social networks, and connections, he elaborated, and the same inputs do not always produce the same outcomes because populations evolve and adapt over time. He added that real populations also display emergent properties—properties that emerge only when individuals interact in a broader population and that are distinct from the properties of each individual or the aggregate of individuals.

Galea described the COVID-19 pandemic's reflection of the true characteristics of populations, pointing out such features as a tremendous diversity in global behaviors, randomness in the location of outbreaks in some urban areas but not others, and the essential role of contact structures and networks in mapping disease transmission. It is truly a picture of a complex system, he observed, emphasizing the importance of addressing such complex public health issues with approaches that go beyond linear, deterministic frameworks.

Turning to discuss obesity, Galea indicated that its exhibiting of classic epidemic behaviors makes it well suited to examination and intervention using systems science approaches. A vast range of inputs contribute to the determination of obesity, he pointed out, recalling the UK Foresight Group's map that Hammond had shared. According to Galea, the map makes it abundantly clear that the only rational way to address obesity is to approach it as a complex system.

Galea shifted to expound on the compatibility of population health with systems thinking by reviewing three of nine principles that have been advanced as foundations of population health science (Keyes and Galea, 2016). The first, he began, is that population health manifests as a continuum. He explained that although this appears obvious, the lack of a simple dichotomy of healthy and unhealthy leads to recognition of the importance of understanding the full spectrum of health within and across populations. As an example, he presented a normal curve distribution of body mass index (BMI) in a population, pointing out that simply providing the proportion of the population that is above the cutoffs for overweight (BMI $\geq 25$ kg/m$^2$) and obesity (BMI $\geq 30$ kg/m$^2$) masks the full scale of distribution of weights and BMIs throughout the population. He asserted that this distribution and the dynamics of its shifts are as or even more important than those proportions. He then showed two overlaid curves illustrating changes in the distribution of BMI between 1976–1980 and 2005–2006 (see Figure 2-2).

Figure 2-2 depicts a more complex shift than that of individuals having (or not having) obesity, Galea emphasized; it demonstrates that the nature of the population curve has changed, which he said requires more sophisticated thinking about the underlying characteristics of the population. He presented another graphic (see Figure 2-3) illustrating the distribution of serum cholesterol levels in men who did or did not develop coronary heart disease in the Framingham Heart Study. Although there was a cutoff cholesterol level above which risk for developing the disease increased,

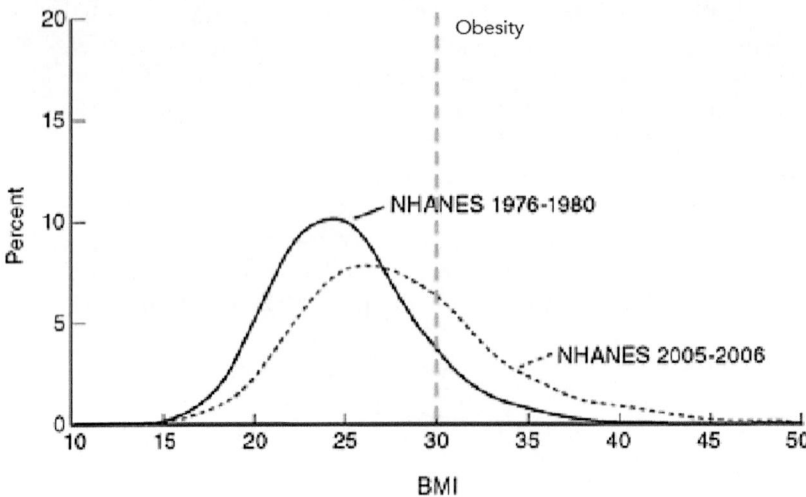

**FIGURE 2-2** Changes in the distribution of body mass index (BMI) between 1976–1980 and 2005–2006 among U.S. adults aged 20–74.
NOTE: NHANES = National Health and Nutrition Examination Survey.
SOURCES: Presented by Sandro Galea, April 6, 2020 (slide 16). Ogden et al., 2007.

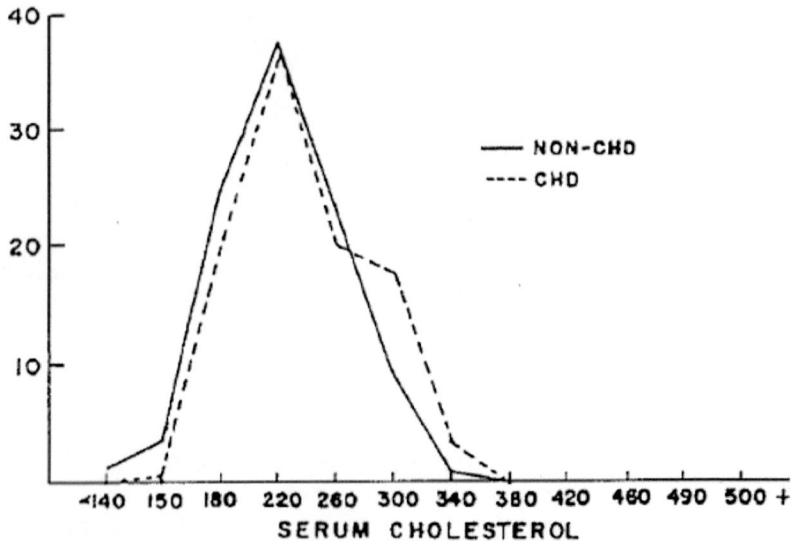

**FIGURE 2-3** Percentage distribution of serum cholesterol levels (milligram/deciliter) in men aged 50–62 who did or did not subsequently develop coronary heart disease (CHD) in the Framingham Heart Study.
SOURCES: Presented by Sandro Galea, April 6, 2020 (slide 17). Rose, 1985.

Galea noted that the curves were quite similar to that point, indicating the importance of understanding the broad factors driving the full shape of the population curve.

Galea moved on to discuss a second foundational principle of population health science: that small changes in ubiquitous causes may result in more substantial change in the health of populations relative to larger changes in rarer causes. He used the metaphor of a goldfish in a fishbowl to illustrate this point. If the goldfish wanted to be healthy, he said, it might receive a variety of behavioral suggestions, such as swimming daily laps and regulating its intake of fish food. But if the water in the bowl—which is ubiquitous around the goldfish—were not changed, such behavioral changes would matter little because the unclean water would hasten its death.

The public tends to think about improving health in a linear, deterministic way, Galea continued, referencing a series of consumer health and fitness books that promote individual behavior changes. He maintained that these books fail to sufficiently consider broader, ubiquitous environmental factors, such as increasing portion sizes of packaged and restaurant foods, which influence and can undermine individual behavior changes. Differences in food environments can help explain heterogeneity in the prevalence of obesity across adjoining communities, he added, and he called for the application of systems science approaches to understand both the individual drivers and the ubiquitous forces that affect population health.

Galea highlighted a third principle: the magnitude of an exposure's effect on disease is dependent on the prevalence of the factors that interact with that exposure. To illustrate this principle, Galea asked workshop participants what percentage of obesity risk is determined by one's genes (the exposure), based on the assumption that only two factors—genes and environment—matter for the outcome. He shared a series of images to simulate two scenarios, one in which the obesogenic environment (i.e., the interacting factor) pervades the entire population and therefore results in obesity among all of the population's genetically predisposed individuals. In this scenario, Galea explained, 100 percent of obesity risk is determined by genes. He described a second scenario with the same population, in which the obesogenic environment affects only a segment of the population. In this scenario, he pointed out, the only genetically predisposed individuals who will develop obesity are those in the segment affected by the obesogenic environment, which in this example is equal to 40 percent of obesity risk determined by genes.

Returning to his question, Galea explained that it is impossible to determine the percentage of obesity risk that is determined by one's genes unless the environment that creates the conditions for the disease is also known. This matters, he continued, because under a plausible assumption of co-occurring causes, the relationship between one cause and the outcome can be understood only if the other cause is also understood. This principle is difficult to grasp, he acknowledged, but he asserted that it is the most fundamental argument for the application of systems thinking to obesity etiology because it accepts that multiple co-occurring factors determine obesity.

Galea moved on to the final portion of his presentation, a discussion of complex systems and counterfactual thinking. He described the concept of a counterfactual by comparing two universes: an observed universe and a parallel universe that is identical to the observed one except for a single variable and the outcome. The observation of a different outcome based on the manipulation of only one variable allows a researcher to determine that the manipulated variable has a causal effect on the outcome, Galea explained, and instills confidence in selecting that variable as the intervention target. He noted that counterfactual theories underlie all of modern causal thinking, but that it is difficult to simulate such parallel universes.

To overcome this difficulty, Galea suggested, systems science approaches can complement observational and experimental techniques to simulate the counterfactual, and although all approaches have imperfections, together they can contribute to a better understanding of strategies for improving population health (Marshall and Galea, 2015). He cautioned against elevating a single approach as the "gold standard." This designation is commonly given to randomized controlled trials (RCTs), he observed, but he asserted that no such "gold standard" exists. Rather, he maintained, the gold standard is a well-designed study that uses appropriate methodologies for the question of interest, articulates its limitations, and offers findings and conclusions that can advance improvement in population health.

Finally, Galea reiterated that principles of population health science illuminate the utility of applying systems thinking to population health issues, but he also urged workshop participants to approach these issues with the mindset of "as simple as possible, but not simpler," a quote attributed to Albert Einstein. In the context of this quote, he recounted a story about John Snow, a pioneer in the field of epidemiology, who convinced local officials to remove the handle of a water pump that he suspected to be the source of a cholera outbreak in London in the mid-1800s. Snow's discovery made a seminal contribution to the understanding of disease transmission, Galea affirmed, but he suggested that this episode in the history of public health has led the public health workforce to a belief in the existence of simple solutions. He contended that it is ineffective to try to simplify solutions by searching for a single cause on which to focus intervention.

In completing his presentation, Galea suggested that the United States has been overly simplistic in its approach to population health, noting its trend of greater health expenditures yet lower life expectancy relative to other high-income countries (Roser, 2017). Population health epidemics such as obesity are driven by a complex set of forces, he stressed. Thus, he called for systems thinking to identify key levers for intervention that will achieve maximal impact to improve overall population health and narrow health inequities.

## APPLICATIONS OF SYSTEMS SCIENCE: CONTEXT, CAUSALITY, AND COMMUNITIES

Douglas Luke, professor and director of the Ph.D. program in public health sciences at Washington University in St. Louis, provided an overview of applications of systems science. Systems science approaches are beneficial for chronic disease prevention and policy implementation, he began, echoing Hammond's and Galea's statements about the complexity of public health problems. He noted that this complexity has led to the coining of the term "wicked problems," which refers to complex problems that resist resolution. He listed characteristics of such problems, including the involvement of multiple actors and sectors, high economic and/or political stakes, interconnectivity with other problems, and lack of agreement or clarity regarding solutions.

Luke shared a causal loop diagram of the complex tobacco landscape (see Figure 2-4), pointing out its heterogeneous, interconnected elements and actors. This complex system cannot be understood by studying its individual parts, he maintained, adding that the important behavior of the system emerges over time when it is examined as a whole. This reality leads to a set of assumptions about the features of complex systems, he explained, including nonlinearity, non-normality, heterogeneity, multiple levels of analysis, and dynamism with feedback. Luke emphasized the interaction of actors in complex systems, and noted that many of the study designs and analytical tools that are typically part of the training of most researchers tend to be poorly suited to addressing this multilevel interaction and heterogeneity.

Luke next described insights related to context, causality, and communities that have stemmed from his group's application of systems science approaches to the study of chronic disease. The first insight, he began, is that these approaches facilitate exploration of the role of context in chronic disease processes. He stated that chronic disease development and interventions are shaped by numerous contextual factors that traditional methods often ignore, yet such problems as obesity cannot be truly understood without considering context. Luke listed important layers of context, including social (both individual and organizational), economic, physical, temporal, and political/historical. It is important to use frameworks or models that capture this rich context, he stressed, noting that the focus is often on specific elements and outcomes of the program, policy, or practice being implemented.

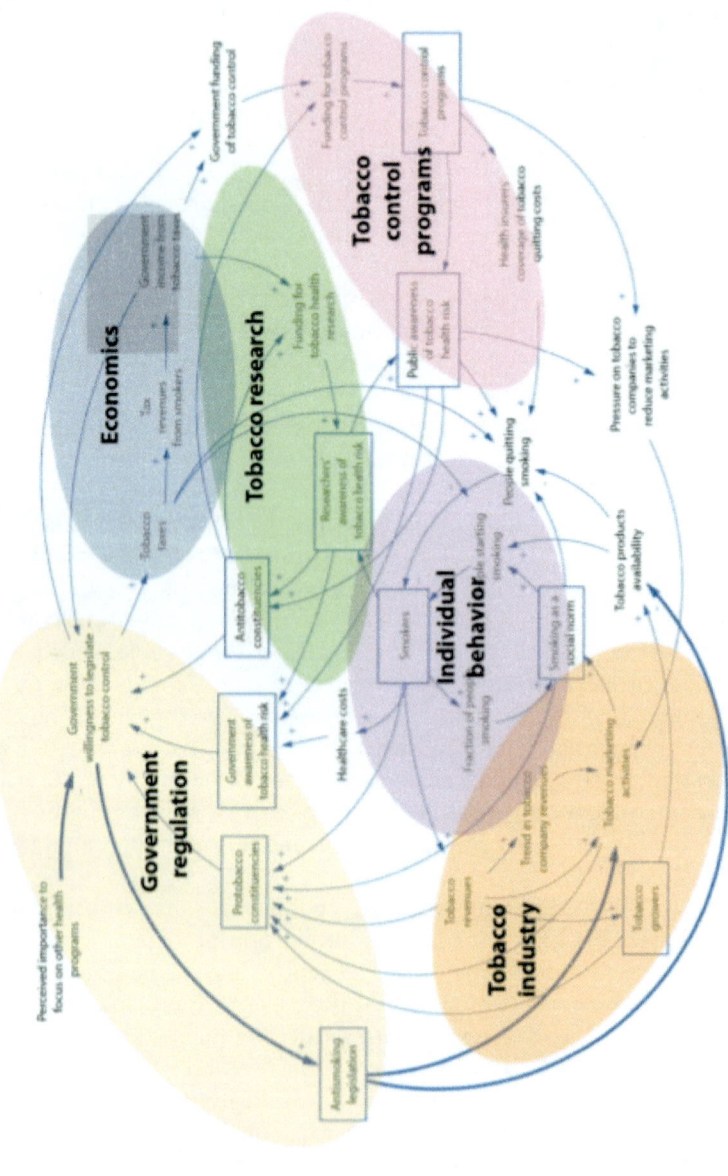

FIGURE 2-4 The complex tobacco landscape.
SOURCES: Presented by Douglas Luke, April 6, 2020. IOM, 2015.

To develop more effective interventions, he suggested, one must understand how they are embedded within higher- and lower-level contexts.

To illustrate this point about the importance of considering context, Luke described a type of traditional epidemiological model that predicts and models the time course of an infectious disease outbreak. An underlying assumption in such a model, he explained, is the average number of contacts per person per unit time, which assumes random mixing and ignores social structures. Nonetheless, this traditional model with its simplifying assumption worked until the 1980s, Luke recounted, when the AIDS epidemic elevated the role of social context in disease transmission. The traditional models were then replaced by network graphics, he continued, which illustrate the nonrandom, social structure of disease transmission (see Figure 2-5). To provide a recent example, Luke described features of a contact tracing network graphic of COVID-19 outbreak clusters in Singapore.[1] He emphasized the importance of physical and social context, such as attending the same church service or traveling on the same airplane flight, in understanding the dynamics of disease transmission.

Luke suggested that this type of analysis is a particularly helpful tool for describing the individual and social contexts for obesity. As an example of social network analysis, he referenced a publication examining the role of peer group structure in smoking initiation among adolescents, highlighting its use of social network analysis to illustrate patterns of peer influence that a regression model would be unlikely to capture (Ennett and Bauman, 1993). As a second example, he cited a series of publications describing the clustering of obesity in personal networks, a phenomenon he said suggests that even noncontagious diseases can be spread through the influence of close social networks and shared environments (Christakis and Fowler, 2007).

Luke went on to observe that network analysis can be extended to map organizational systems, a point he illustrated by referencing a map of a national network of agencies that collaborate to provide tobacco control services and resources for LGBTQ communities (see Figure 2-6). This map illustrates that many of the agencies are connected only through the lead agency (i.e., direct, separate lines from each agency to the lead agency) he pointed out, which he said alerted the funder that additional interorganizational ties would make the system more robust and resistant to network collapse if the lead agency were compromised. Organizational and social systems mapping is also useful for designing interventions or implementing new best practices in clinical settings, Luke added, settings in which interpersonal interactions are important.

Luke then discussed a second insight—that systems science approaches facilitate the exploration of underlying causal mechanisms. He explained

---

[1] See https://www.againstcovid19.com/singapore/cases/search (accessed September 16, 2020).

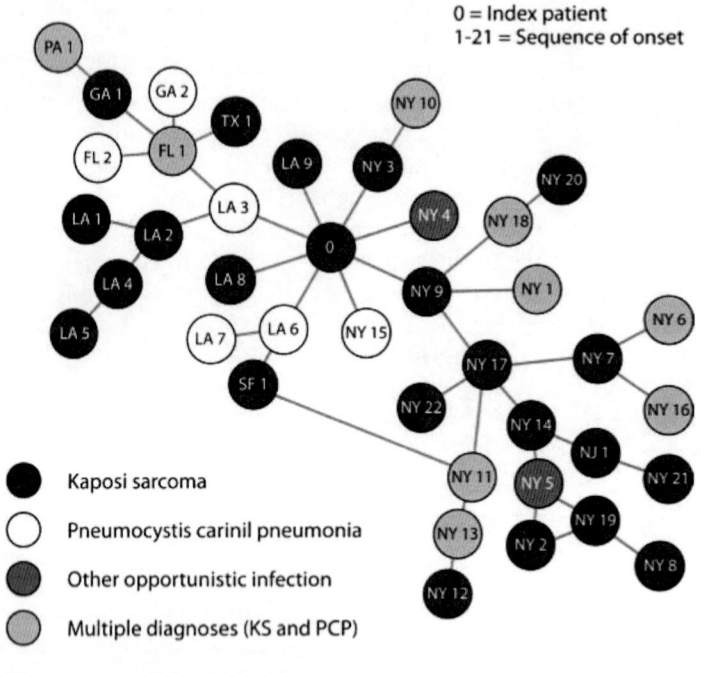

**FIGURE 2-5** The first AIDS network graphic.
SOURCES: Presented by Douglas Luke, April 6, 2020. Auerbach et al., 1984; Luke and Stamatakis, 2012.

that although traditional methods such as RCTs are useful for establishing causality—that is, *whether* something works—they are less useful for determining *how* or *why* something works. He referenced a seminal paper describing numerous uses of computational systems models in public health and societal contexts beyond predicting disease mortality, such as illuminating dynamics central to the system at hand and suggesting analogous dynamics within other systems (Epstein, 2008).

To illustrate how complex systems models can help identify the inner workings of underlying causal mechanisms, Luke described Tobacco Town, a modeling effort from his policy research on tobacco control. Tobacco Town, which uses the systems science approach of agent-based modeling, is a policy laboratory used to explore potential impacts of various retail policies across contexts and populations. Luke explained that Tobacco Town is based on evidence indicating that people who live in neighborhoods with a high density of tobacco retailers are more likely to start smoking and

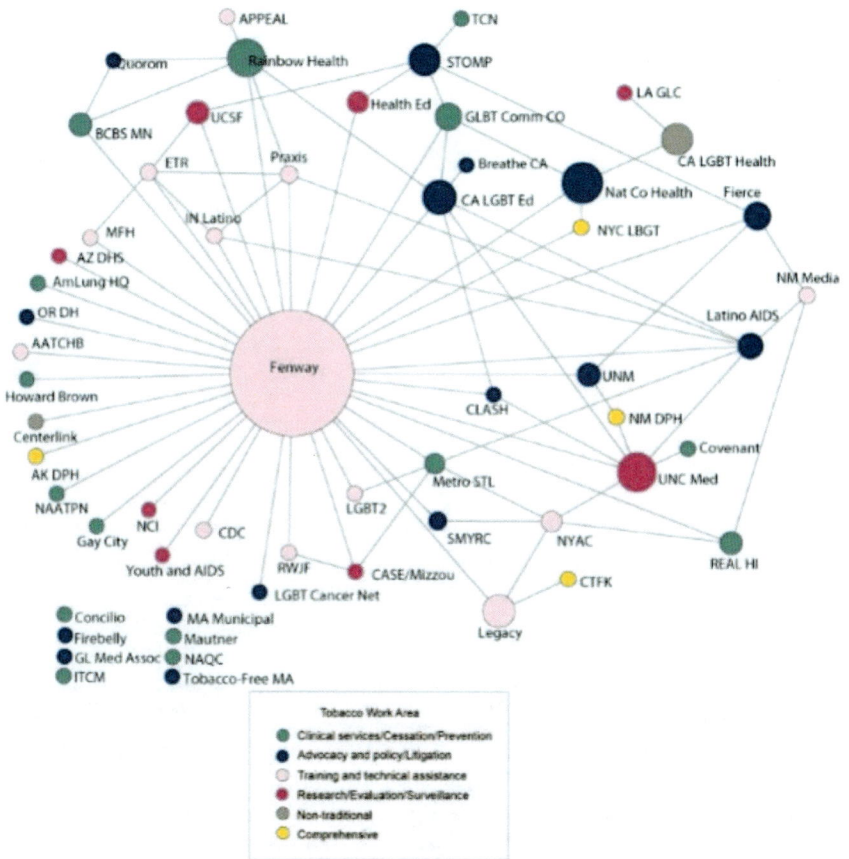

**FIGURE 2-6** Example of an organizational systems map.
SOURCE: Presented by Douglas Luke, April 6, 2020.

have difficulty quitting. The logical policy response would be to reduce the density of tobacco retailers, he continued, but such reduction is difficult to study in the real world. Different communities take different actions at different times, he explained, and clarity is lacking about how density reduction would work in practice.

Luke's research team developed a "mechanism metaphor," he recounted, starting with the assumption of a simple linear relationship whereby a high density of tobacco retailers lowers the time and monetary costs of obtaining tobacco products (see Figure 2-7). He described a mental model in which a sample tobacco user lives in a dense, urban environment. This person does not have to travel far to purchase tobacco, he pointed out, and her behavior is unlikely to change if only one or even a few retailers in a given

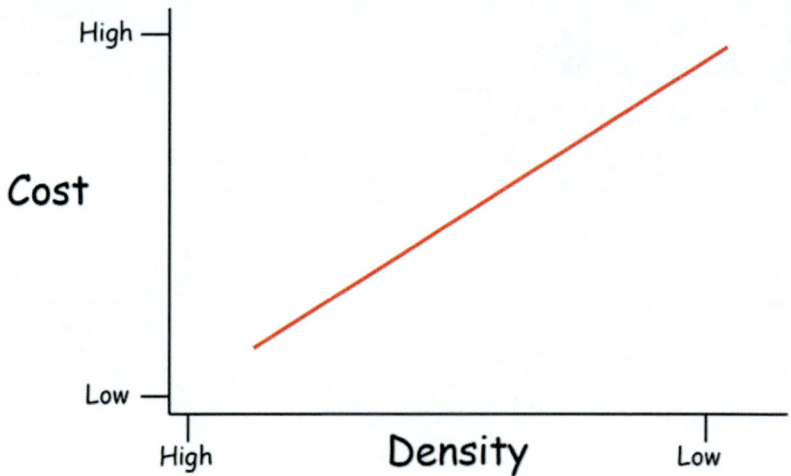

**FIGURE 2-7** Assumed linear relationship between density of tobacco retailers and time and monetary costs of procuring tobacco products.
SOURCE: Presented by Douglas Luke, April 6, 2020.

intersection are removed. Only when she has to travel farther to purchase tobacco is she likely to notice that the density of retailers has been reduced.

Luke identified as one implication of this mental model that the assumption of linearity is likely false; instead, there is likely a nonlinear or threshold effect. Another implication, he continued, is that tobacco-seeking behaviors and any interventions designed to influence them are environmentally dependent, so Tobacco Town entails building computer-based, virtual towns as simulation models to identify interactions between the retail tobacco environment and purchase and use behaviors. Researchers collaborate with community stakeholders to tailor models to specific communities, he elaborated, so they can test the impact of policies prioritized by community members and disseminate the results.

Luke reviewed examples of Tobacco Town in action to show that it confirmed the nonlinearity between retailer density and the costs of procuring tobacco products. Reduction of retailer density may need to reach a threshold, he explained, before behavior effects are observed. The patterns of these effects differ based on the urbanicity and income levels of modeled towns, he added, an observation that implies that policies have different potential for affecting disparities and behaviors in different types of communities.

Luke shared a heat map visualization of the potential effects of two types of tobacco retailer policies as an example of how agent-based modeling can facilitate the exploration of underlying mechanisms. One policy requires a 600-meter buffer between retailers, while the other requires a 600-meter buffer between retailers and schools. Luke explained that, when applied to the city of Philadelphia, the first policy reduced retailer density from 4.5 to 0.6 retailers per square kilometer and increased the average distance between residents and retailers from 200 to 480 kilometers. By contrast, he said, the second policy reduced retailer density from 4.5 to 0.76 retailers per square kilometer and increased the average distance between residents and retailers from 200 to 730 kilometers. Luke pointed out that although the resulting retailer density metric looks similar for both policies, the second policy has a greater impact on proximity because it creates a much higher average distance between residents and retailers. According to Luke, the underlying mechanism of proximity in this example has implications for community policy development and intervention.

Luke then outlined three advantages of such mechanism-based modeling. First, understanding how a policy works opens the door to designing more effective policies or interventions with less guesswork; second, it helps stakeholders advocate more persuasively for programs to be maintained or terminated; and third, it offers a new way to understand health disparities by focusing on the processes through which those disparities arise, rather than simply documenting them.

Luke's third insight was that systems science approaches can produce tools that are highly relevant and useful for community stakeholders and policy makers. He revisited the paper he had mentioned previously to list three additional uses of computational systems models: training practitioners, disciplining the policy dialogue, and educating the public (Epstein, 2008). To illustrate this third insight, he recalled an application of the Tobacco Town model to communities in Minnesota where the effects of policies to reduce the density of tobacco retailers depended on context. Baseline retailer density varied by community urbanicity (rural, suburban, or urban) and income level (high or low), he elaborated, and the Tobacco Town dashboard illustrated how various policies would potentially affect retailer density across these different types of communities. He noted that as policies became stronger, to include restricting tobacco sales at pharmacies and requiring buffers between retailers, retailer density dropped considerably in all communities, and disparities in density diminished across communities of varying urbanicity and income levels.

In a final example of disseminating systems science tools to community stakeholders, Luke showed workshop participants an interactive Tobacco Swamp dashboard his group is developing to help policy makers explore the effects—based on underlying computational models—of different retailer-focused tobacco control policies in different cities. He loaded Washington,

DC, into the dashboard[2] as an example, and observed that nearly 100 percent of its residents are within a 10-minute walk of a tobacco retailer. As he selected various policy interventions in the dashboard, he pointed out how the different options, such as school buffers, could be expected to affect retailer density in the city.

## PANEL DISCUSSION

Rivera moderated a panel discussion with the three session speakers following their presentations. Topics addressed included the importance of applying systems science approaches to obesity solutions and potential metrics of success; examples of communicating systems science concepts to academics, policy makers, and the public; the role of leadership and the alignment of multisector action in systems science approaches; the types of training and collaboration that can help prepare stakeholders to undertake systems modeling efforts; and funding opportunities for systems science approaches.

### Importance of Applying Systems Science
### Approaches and Metrics of Success

Rivera began by asking the speakers to explain why it is critical to apply a systems science approach to obesity solutions and to describe how they would measure success in doing so during the next 5 years. Hammond reiterated the importance of implementing packages of interventions to address the obesity epidemic, an approach he said is inherently systems-focused because it calls on stakeholders to assemble different packages for different settings and to coordinate efforts into a coherent set of solutions. He voiced his 5-year vision for progress in blending systems science tools with conventional tools to create a package of actions and processes that communities can leverage to tackle obesity as they apply this package to their specific context and evidence base.

Galea agreed that obesity solutions are not one size fits all, and emphasized the importance of identifying the highest-priority factors to address in a particular place at a given point in time. Different contexts call for different sets of solutions, he argued, cautioning against deterministic perspectives that simplify problems and apply the same approach across the board. He suggested that an indication of success would be the use of sophisticated thinking to assemble a suite of context- and time-specific approaches to obesity solutions in communities.

---

[2] See https://aspirecenter.org/tobacco-swamps (accessed October 20, 2020).

Luke commented on the difference between efficacy and effectiveness, noting that although an intervention's success may be predicted under ideal conditions, its real-world outcome can be quite different. The difference is often systemic in nature, he suggested, giving the example of a real-world tobacco retail policy that generates responses from industry and retailers. Such effects are sometimes called unintended consequences, Luke added, but he noted that some systems science models reject this term and simply call them consequences.

## Communicating Systems Science Concepts to Academics, Policy Makers, and the Public

Rivera next asked the speakers to share examples of an effective explanation of systems science concepts to academics, policy makers, and the public. Hammond acknowledged that different strategies for communicating with each of these audiences are often warranted, but stated that data visualization tools are useful for explaining systems science models to both policy makers and the public. Visualizations can convey sophisticated dynamics without complex data tables and equations, he elaborated, and can communicate powerfully as they portray location- and context-specific scenarios. As for academics and scientists, Hammond suggested that they are interested in whether systems science models yield insights and results that might have been unattainable with other techniques.

Galea suggested a paradox in that scientists may find it more difficult to grasp systems science approaches because academic training tends to guide doctoral students to narrow their expertise to a particular exposure and outcome. Conversely, he said, systems science approaches have intuitive appeal for policy makers and the public, although he warned that such methods as agent-based modeling can lead policy makers to have false confidence in the ability to predict future outcomes. The communication challenge for modelers, he argued, is to explain the utility of these models alongside their caveats and limitations. Luke concurred, urging researchers to be "appropriately skeptical" about a model's capabilities when they discuss using modeled results to plan action with community stakeholders.

## The Role of Leadership and Alignment of Multisector Action

Rivera asked the speakers to discuss the role of leadership and the alignment of multisector action based on systems science approaches. Galea referenced epidemiologist Geoffrey Rose's declaration that it is not population health scientists' role to determine action; rather, their role is to present options and let policy makers balance various inputs to determine the appropriate action. As an example, he noted that many infectious disease models publicized during the COVID-19 pandemic have been used to determine blunt policy approaches. This is inappropriate, Galea asserted, and he urged that leaders avoid "model absolutism" by considering a full spectrum of potential consequences—including those forecast by models and those not modeled—in light of various societal values and the moral and philosophical worldviews that underlie them. Models are "vastly imperfect," he stressed, a limitation that he said elevates the role of leadership in balancing both modeled and nonmodeled inputs.

Hammond emphasized that models are just one of many inputs for decision making and do not replace the need for judgment or eliminate uncertainty. He suggested that models could be more useful for decision making if stakeholders and decision makers were engaged early in their development and use. He also pointed to MIDAS as a network including multiple models that are developed by different groups and can be communicated as an ensemble to policy makers. He shared a lesson from the 2009–2010 H1N1 pandemic: the importance of having a "translator" who understands the abilities and limitations of models and is conversant in the vernacular of both modelers and policy makers. This role can bridge the two worlds, he explained, and help prevent problems that could otherwise arise.

Luke concurred in urging that systems modeling efforts be multidisciplinary and transdisciplinary from the beginning, including modelers, subject-matter experts, translators, and community stakeholders and decision makers. He recounted past efforts that failed to incorporate these perspectives, which he said turned out to be a poor use of resources.

Hammond highlighted the importance of training, explaining that systems models are relatively easy to use poorly if not applied and interpreted properly. The skills of modeling and computer programming are distinct, he said, explaining that the former involves discerning what variables and assumptions to include and how to engage with the right stakeholders.

### Training and Collaboration

Rivera asked the speakers to elaborate on the types of training and collaboration that can help prepare stakeholders to undertake systems modeling efforts. Hammond underscored that substantial training and experience are essential to the appropriate use of systems science tools. He called for training that provides learners with a sophisticated understanding of the tools' capabilities and limitations so they can participate effectively in teams that include modeling experts. He added that to become a full-fledged modeling practitioner, a multiyear investment is expected, typically in the context of a doctoral program or apprenticeship.

Luke remarked that the environment for training opportunities has improved over the past few years. He mentioned a summer institute that he conducts with Hammond at Washington University in St. Louis to provide an introduction to predominant systems science approaches that enhance the social impact of health and social science research. An impetus for the institute, he explained, was that many of their research partners lacked access to full doctoral-level classes in systems science approaches.

Galea agreed that it takes dedication to develop the expertise necessary to use systems science approaches effectively. He also emphasized the importance of participating in transdisciplinary teams so that population health stakeholders can engage with expert modelers. Luke concurred with the value of a team-based approach, noting that all members need not be expert modelers. He added that systems science training often emphasizes systems science methodologies, but not systems thinking. Galea agreed, and cautioned against blindly using a particular method without contemplating whether it is being used to ask the right questions.

Rivera commented that transdisciplinary efforts had become more common over the course of his career. When problems are discussed among transdisciplinary collaborators, he observed, their diverse mindsets can initially breed tension, but as they are exposed to different ways of thinking about the problem at hand, these initial mindsets evolve and a shared vocabulary develops, allowing everyone to understand the problem better. Hammond described systems modeling as a journey rather than a destination and provided two examples to support his point. First, he explained that some of the most valuable contributions to modeling come from the process of documenting mental models. This process includes providing data that support the model's assumptions, Hammond elaborated, and is aided by qualitative and quantitative tools that help one think like a modeler. Second, he continued, models are often iterative. The success of such groups as MIDAS, he observed, is based on sustained investment that allowed such iteration to occur and the questions, data, and assumptions that feed into models to be refined, making them better.

## Funding Opportunities

Rivera invited the speakers to share funding opportunities for the use of systems science approaches. Galea and Luke reported a gradually improving landscape with regard to funders' recognition of the value of incorporating these approaches into federally funded research on public health topics. Luke observed that NIH's review committees are increasingly including members with modeling expertise, and Hammond suggested that increased training will grow the pool of experts who can fill reviewer roles. Funding opportunities for systems science approaches have been limited, Hammond suggested, by the relatively small set of experts who are qualified to review proposals that include these approaches. Another limitation, he said, is the relatively long time horizon required to iterate and fine-tune systems efforts, which has implications for the types of funding vehicles and teams that are assembled.

## AUDIENCE DISCUSSION

Following the panel discussion, speakers addressed questions from workshop participants about mapping systems components, building community capacity to use models and propel policy change, lessons learned from the transportation sector, funding mechanisms to support systems science approaches, and training physicians in health systems science.

### Approaches to Mapping Systems Components

In response to a question about approaches to mapping complex systems in order to identify relevant features and processes, Galea replied that when stakeholders review a base of literature as part of the modeling process, they identify parameters that can inform models, as well as areas in which literature does not exist to inform other parameters. This identification of gaps leads to proposing studies that can fill these gaps, he observed, or to articulating the ranges of assumptions that will be included in a model.

According to Hammond, participatory group model building is a qualitative systems science approach that can engage community members and stakeholders in articulating their lived experiences in systems. Tapping into community members' perspectives and experiences can help researchers better understand and visualize systems structures, he explained, adding that the translation of these qualitative inputs into quantitative models must be done carefully.

Luke noted that systems science approaches can be used to inform theories and meet community needs. He pointed out that systems mapping, an approach that uses network methods to examine the organizational interconnections in a community, helps provide a springboard for a community's future research, evaluation, and planning.

### Building Community Capacity to Use Models and Propel Policy Change

Luke emphasized that it is important for researchers to understand community partners' perspectives on the research. They must explain clearly why community partners should care about the work, he maintained, and this can be accomplished by involving them from the outset. He referenced his colleague Ross Brownson's concept of "designing for dissemination," which entails thinking about dissemination at the start of a project.

In response to a question about how to use systems maps to drive policy change, Luke replied that resources are available online with which communities can test different scenarios. Researchers may get face time with community partners, he added, but virtual technologies provide access to partners around the world. Most online resources are open-access and easily available, Luke continued, and some sustainability assessment tools have been released under the Creative Commons license. It takes expertise to develop dashboards that are user-friendly in the way they present results and allow stakeholder interaction, he noted, calling out R Shiny products as helpful for that purpose.

Luke explained that his group developed its Tobacco Town models in close consultation with a variety of community and policy partners to increase the models' potential for community impact. He highlighted the value of working with legal experts to help shape how potential tobacco control policies are presented, given that they may be contested in court over First Amendment or other constitutional challenges.

## Lessons Learned from the Transportation Sector

Models have been used to inform urban development, Luke said, such as by incorporating data on travel patterns to aid in improving traffic congestion. Rivera observed that transportation modeling efforts tap into a plethora of GPS and other contextual data (e.g., from satellite radio) to generate their results. He suggested that using these sources of contextual data would improve understanding of obesity as well. Hammond pointed out that in any sector, policy decision making involves trade-offs between various outcomes of interest, and that models can help optimize different policy objectives.

## Funding Mechanisms to Support Systems Science Approaches

Luke observed that some systems science approaches, such as group model building and network mapping, require less time and money than others. Therefore, he reasoned, it would be useful to have a variety of funding opportunities to support different types of systems science approaches. In the context of obesity, Hammond suggested that funding opportunities incentivize the formation of interdisciplinary teams with heterogeneous expertise in methods and content, ideally across institutions and geographies. According to Hammond, some grant development mechanisms, such as the NIH process, are generally not well suited to this objective, and a funding mechanism to ensure such interdisciplinary collaboration would need to be carefully crafted. Galea advocated for including junior investigators in these collaborations to create a pipeline of scholars who naturally engage in systems thinking.

## Training Physicians in Health Systems Science

A workshop participant stated that health systems science is now considered the third pillar of medicine, joining basic and clinical science, and asked the speakers how future physicians could be trained to understand the role of human factors, systems engineering, leadership, and patient improvement strategies so as to transform health care and ensure greater patient safety. Galea said he was happy to hear that systems thinking is entering medical school curricula, noting that it is important for physicians to recognize that a complex set of determinants drives patients' clinical outcomes. He cautioned against charging physicians with solving the complex systems problems that ultimately shape population health, noting that their primary role is to provide clinical care, which is only one component of broader systems. Hammond agreed, and added that systems science approaches can be used to study and make changes in the health care system.

## CLOSING REMARKS FOR PART I

Following the discussion, Christina Economos, co-founder and director of ChildObesity180 and professor and New Balance chair in childhood nutrition at the Friedman School of Nutrition Science, Tufts University, recapped key points from Part I of the workshop:

- Systems science approaches and systems thinking can be used in concert with traditional research designs and approaches. This implies that there is benefit in interdisciplinary collaboration involving trained teams of community stakeholders, translators, modelers, and scientists.
- Contextual effects are important and can be measured if they are considered in analyses and captured with dynamic, real-time data.
- Real-world experiments are costly and time-intensive, but systems science approaches using quantitative and qualitative methods allow for tailoring and testing of multilevel solutions and policies—such as those that address health inequities—in specific communities, populations, and contexts.
- Advances in data visualization have helped communicate the outputs of systems science approaches, demonstrating the value of these approaches and making them more accessible to scientists, practitioners, policy makers, trainees, and the public.

# 3

# Complex Systems in Society and the Context for Obesity

---

**Highlights from the Presentations of Individual Speakers**

- Systems science approaches can illuminate racism-related dimensions of obesity morbidity and mortality. Critical race theory can help systems science approaches identify underlying racial drivers of obesity and associated inequities by incorporating racism in mental models and analyses, addressing racialized power dynamics, and addressing the social construction of knowledge. (Chandra Ford)
- Adults and children with obesity tend to cluster in social networks, and having social connections with obesity increases a person's obesity risk over time. Therefore, much potential exists to leverage social networks as part of a systems science approach to solutions for obesity. (Kayla de la Haye)
- Systems science approaches are well suited to examining neighborhood effects on health because of their utility for understanding the bidirectional person–environment relations that occur in neighborhoods, as well as their ability to parse interactions among people, interactions and interrelations between physical and social environments, and spatial patterning (i.e., segregation) of individual and environmental characteristics. (Ana Diez Roux)
- Agent-based modeling that simulated the impact of crime on physical activity and obesity among Black women in

---

> Washington, DC, revealed that as an individual's propensity to exercise increased, reductions in crime that increased the accessibility of locations for physical activity were associated with a greater decrease in the prevalence of obesity. (Tiffany Powell-Wiley)

Part II of the workshop began with a session exploring complex systems in society that provide the context for obesity and have the potential to shape population health and well-being. Shiriki Kumanyika, emerita professor of epidemiology at the University of Pennsylvania Perelman School of Medicine and research professor in the Department of Community Health & Prevention at the Dornsife School of Public Health, Drexel University, moderated the first half of the session, during which two speakers discussed power dynamics, structural racism, and relationships. Giselle Corbie-Smith, the Kenan Distinguished Professor and director of the Center for Health Equity Research at the University of North Carolina at Chapel Hill, moderated the second half of the session, during which two additional speakers discussed resources, place-based issues, policy, and political will.

## POWER DYNAMICS AND STRUCTURAL RACISM: INSIGHTS FROM CRITICAL RACE THEORY

Chandra Ford, associate professor of community health sciences and founding director of the Center for the Study of Racism, Social Justice & Health at the University of California, Los Angeles, discussed power dynamics and structural racism from the lens of critical race theory (CRT). She began by noting that she conducts her work on lands originally inhabited by the Tongva people, which, she said, shows that even those fighting for racial equity are complicit with and benefit from the historical and ongoing injustices to which indigenous peoples of the Americas have been subjected.

Ford began by drawing a parallel between systems science approaches, which help uncover complex relationships among systems that contribute to morbidity and mortality, and CRT, which she said draws on sophisticated conceptual and empirical approaches to identify and explain otherwise imperceptible racial drivers of inequities in society. She quoted Camara Jones's (2000) definition of racism as "a system of structuring opportunity and assigning value based on the social interpretation of how one looks that unfairly disadvantages some individuals and communities, unfairly advantages other individuals and communities, and saps the strength of the whole society through the waste of human resources." According to Ford, nuanced forms of racism remain entrenched and effective at sustaining racial inequities.

CRT, Ford continued, originated with legal scholars of color in the late 1980s as a set of intellectual ideas, principles, and approaches to identifying, understanding, and undoing the root causes of racial hierarchies as they operate in the post–civil rights era. Critical race theorists ask how racism is relevant to a project, Ford explained, and to the production of knowledge about a problem. She highlighted several founding critical race theorists: Derrick Bell, who asserted that to address the less perceptible forms of racism, their mechanisms must first be made explicit through racism-conscious research; Kimberlé Crenshaw, who coined the term "intersectionality" to explain the presence of multiple overlapping, interacting social group identities (such as being both Black and low-income) that have synergistic effects on an individual's risks and cannot be disentangled; and Cheryl Harris, who promulgated the concept of whiteness as property, which maintains that "holders" of whiteness have the same privileges and benefits accorded holders of other types of property. Ford briefly mentioned a model for applying CRT to the health sciences—Public Health Critical Race Praxis—which she described as an offshoot of CRT (Ford and Airhihenbuwa, 2010a,b, 2018).

Ford moved on to explain that models are imperfect representations of reality and that most systematically overlook the primacy of racialization. She suggested three ways in which CRT can help obesity-focused systems science approaches address these constraints. She cited first identifying and incorporating racism in mental models and analyses. Substantial evidence links racism to health, she maintained, and system dynamics models that include appropriate measures of racism could illuminate how structural racism contributes to obesity. She provided several resources[1] for measuring racism at the individual, institutional, and socioecological levels, and urged measurement of race and ethnicity as social constructs. "Races" are not absolute entities, Ford asserted, elaborating that racialized groups exist relative to one another and that race is a differentiating trait that serves as a social mechanism for producing groups and hierarchies. She suggested that focusing on social construction indicates the importance of assessing (1) perceived versus self-reported race, noting that the latter might differ from identity; and (2) how gender, ethnicity, and other factors may inform both perceived and reported identity. She briefly noted that ethnicity is also a social construct and that strategies exist for measuring it as such.

Ford's second suggestion for helping systems science approaches better represent reality was to address racialized power dynamics. She identified community-based participatory research as an approach that has encouraged equitable partnerships between researchers and communities as an

---

[1] Racism: Science & Tools for the Public Health Professional. See https://ajph.aphapublications.org/doi/book/10.2105/9780875533049 (accessed September 11, 2020).

ethical and sustainable path to health equity. Power sharing will become more important in a systems science environment, Ford stressed, to the extent that the environment enables researchers to access more information about communities than communities can access themselves. Racism is embedded in some sources of big data, she argued, and big data may be used in ways that reinforce racial or ethnic marginalization (e.g., Benjamin, 2019; Noble, 2018). To illustrate this point, she observed that surveillance mechanisms disproportionately target people of color for criminal, social, and other forms of policing, and that systems may share data about individuals in communities without involving or seeking consent from those communities. She pointed out that social movements, such as Data for Black Lives,[2] are emerging to challenge these practices, with the objectives of limiting surveillance of communities and democratizing access to data.

Ford's third suggestion for improving systems science approaches was to address the social construction of knowledge. She elaborated by quoting sociologist Lawrence Bobo (2004): "Data never speak for themselves. It is the questions we pose (and those we fail to ask) as well as our theories, concepts, and ideas that bring a narrative and meaning to marginal distributions, correlations, regression coefficients, and statistics of all kinds." Ford went on to note that although the scientific method enhances the reliability of empirical findings, it does not necessarily eliminate the influence of racial bias (Ford and Airhihenbuwa, 2018).

Ford suggested that researchers engage in "critical reflexivity" to assess how they may apply inadvertent subjectivity to their work. She explained this process by describing the Human Immunodeficiency Virus Testing, Linkage and Retention in care (HIV TLR) study (Ford et al., 2018). This 5-year retrospective cohort study linked multiple large datasets to electronic medical records, she explained, to examine contextual determinants of racial/ethnic disparities in outcomes along the HIV care continuum in Southern California. Each member of the study team completed a confidential questionnaire prior to each new arm, Ford explained, that assessed the member's expected results, the level of certainty about each prediction, the nature of any expected disparities, and the basis for those expectations. The purpose of the questionnaire was to understand whether team members were inclined to endorse potential results that aligned with their a priori assumptions. According to Ford, the results indicated that raising people's awareness of their biases and increasing the amount of time they have to respond to those biases may reduce the biases' inadvertent effects.

Based on her broader experience in this area, Ford listed five questions that could potentially guide the next steps for applying systems science approaches to obesity efforts:

---

[2] See https://d4bl.org (accessed October 9, 2020).

- What are best practices for sharing power with communities in a systems science approach?
- What racial biases are embedded in the data on which systems science approaches rely?
- How does the (uncritical) use of such data reinforce the marginalization of communities of color (e.g., via surveillance)?
- How might racialization/racism affect biological systems?
- To what extent are relational gains for the dominant racial group (i.e., Whites) obscured even in work on disparities?

Ford closed by stating that systems science approaches hold promise for tackling the complex phenomenon of obesity, and that these approaches can illuminate racism-related dimensions of the morbidity and mortality associated with obesity. Racism pervades every societal system, she maintained, although its greatest impacts are difficult to perceive, and she argued that CRT can help systems science approaches identify underlying racial drivers of obesity and associated inequities.

## SOCIAL NETWORKS AND RELATIONSHIPS

Kayla de la Haye, assistant professor of preventive medicine at the University of Southern California, prefaced her presentation on social networks and relationships by referencing the difficulty of changing eating and activity habits. A triangular relapse pattern is well known in obesity interventions, she said, whereby people who can access and adhere to evidence-based interventions often cannot sustain their initial modifications in lifestyle behaviors (see Figure 3-1). This pattern may occur, de la Haye explained, because people are able to exert personal agency, choice, and effort toward behavior change at the outset of an intervention, but they are not embedded in social and environmental structures that support healthful habits over the long term. She stressed that people with low incomes and communities of color are unequally exposed to structural influences that do not support healthful habits; therefore, interventions need to target multiple factors across layers of individual, social, physical, and macro-environmental systems that influence obesity risk.

de la Haye suggested that much potential exists to leverage social environments, particularly the rich social networks that make up social fabrics, in systems science solutions for obesity. These include local social networks of family, friends, and community contacts that can influence obesity risk (see Figure 3-2), she elaborated, as well as global social networks of community members, stakeholders, and decision makers that shape the structural features of lived environments. She clarified her definition of "social networks" as denoting social structures comprising social actors and their

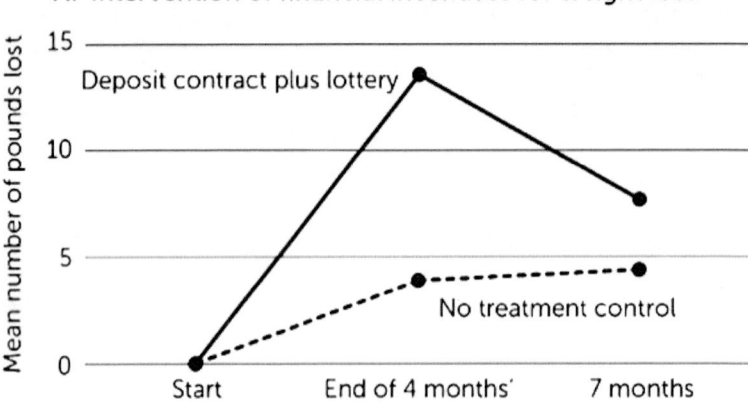

FIGURE 3-1 The triangular relapse pattern in health behavior change over time.
SOURCES: Presented by Kayla de la Haye, June 30, 2020. Wood and Neal, 2016.

interrelationships. These networks, she explained, transcend the online space and represent diverse types of relationships and social actors, such as kinship or friendship among community members; collaboration among organizations; or even partnerships among cities, states, and countries. She added that they are often illustrated with nodes representing social actors and with lines or ties between the nodes representing relationships that can have many different qualities.

Next, de la Haye described social network analysis, a broad theoretical and analytic framework used to study emergent patterns of actors and ties in a network, such as by identifying the occupants of knowledge-brokering positions that link disconnected communities and determining which social actors share close and clustered connections. As an example, she pointed to the use of social network analysis to study the racial and ethnic underpinnings of friendship network structures in high schools or the patterns of collaboration among different types of member organizations in a community coalition.

Social network analysis is also used to study the impact of social structures on individual and group outcomes, de la Haye continued, referencing research indicating that adults and children with obesity tend to cluster in social networks and that social connections with obesity increase a person's obesity risk over time. She added that longitudinal research has linked these patterns to several contributing factors, which include homophily, propinquity, and stigma (see Figure 3-3). Homophily is a phenomenon whereby people tend to select or form social ties with others who have similar

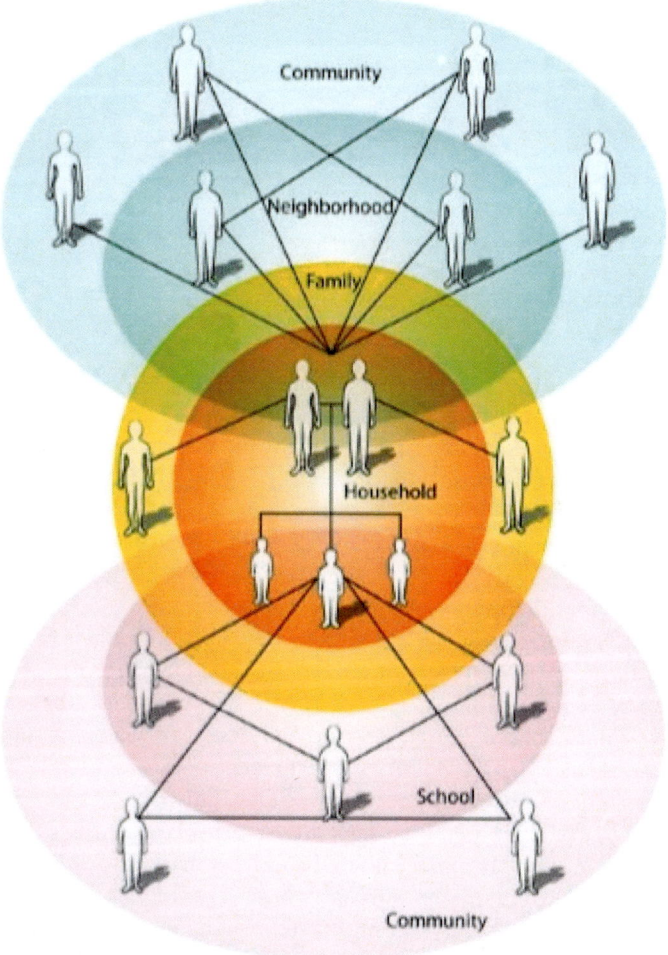

FIGURE 3-2 Example of local, personal social networks with the potential to influence obesity risk.
SOURCES: Presented by Kayla de la Haye, June 30, 2020. Koehly and Loscalzo, 2009.

characteristics, de la Haye explained, such as ethnicity, socioeconomic status, or health risks and inequalities (Centola, 2011; de la Haye et al., 2011; Schaefer and Simpkins, 2014; Schaefer et al., 2011; Valente et al., 2009). Propinquity, she went on, refers to people connecting to others through shared social and physical spaces in homes, communities, and organizations, where structural and environmental influences are similar. Weight-based stigma is a third driver of these patterns of obesity in social networks, she

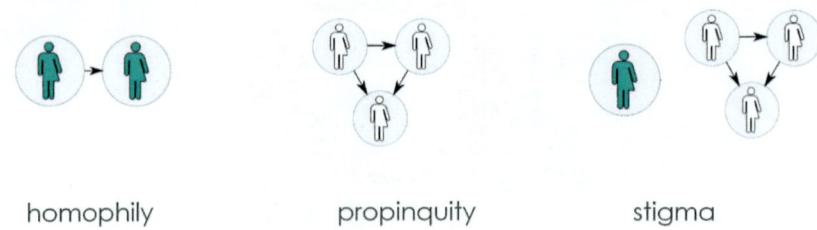

homophily                          propinquity                          stigma

**FIGURE 3-3** Factors that contribute to the clustering of obesity in social networks.
SOURCE: Presented by Kayla de la Haye, June 30, 2020.

said, explaining that people with obesity are often socially rejected by peers who do not have obesity. Over time, she continued, this phenomenon results in the formation of more social connections among individuals with similar weight status and marginalization of those who have overweight.

In addition to those three drivers, de la Haye explained, evidence indicates that social ties directly influence people's weight norms and weight-related behaviors through a number of social influence mechanisms, which can lead to similarities in the risks for overweight among family members and friends (Aral and Nicolaides, 2017; de la Haye et al., 2011; Hammond et al., 2012; Simpkins et al., 2011; Trogdon et al., 2008; Valente et al., 2009; Zhang et al., 2018). Resource support and social capital within networks can also impact obesity risk, she added, citing a study of the personal networks of Mexican American adults that found that having more health support in one's personal social network predicted better diet quality, especially for people experiencing food insecurity (Flórez et al., 2020).[3]

Overall, de la Haye summarized, these dynamics of social selection, social influence, and corresponding shared exposures give rise to the clustering of obesity that researchers have observed in social networks. This observation highlights a critical feedback loop and intervention target, she pointed out, because people at high risk of developing obesity and impacted by inequities are more likely to find themselves in social networks that also confer health risks, and that influence and exacerbate people's future risk for obesity.

In the final portion of her presentation, de la Haye shared examples of intervention approaches designed to leverage or change social networks as part of obesity solutions. She highlighted segmentation as one common strategy for local social networks, an approach that targets at-risk social groups (e.g., family or peer groups) rather than individuals for collective

---

[3] See http://www.pfeffer.at/sunbelt/talks/1142.html (accessed December 1, 2020).

behavior change and as promoters of positive social influence, norms, and support for healthy habits (Valente, 2012). As a second strategy she cited alteration, in which an intervention aims to change people's social networks by building new, adjacent health networks that can increase access to positive social influences, norms, and support (Valente, 2012).

Next, de la Haye described the application of both segmentation and alteration in an intervention called Healthy Home, Healthy Habits that she and her colleagues designed and are evaluating (de la Haye et al., 2019). This intervention, she explained, aims to promote healthy dietary and activity habits for low-income mothers and their infants while simultaneously creating healthy changes in the home environment and creating new social ties among mothers in the program through group-based interventions and activities that seek to build meaningful and lasting social connections (see Figure 3-4). The intervention also connects mothers to community

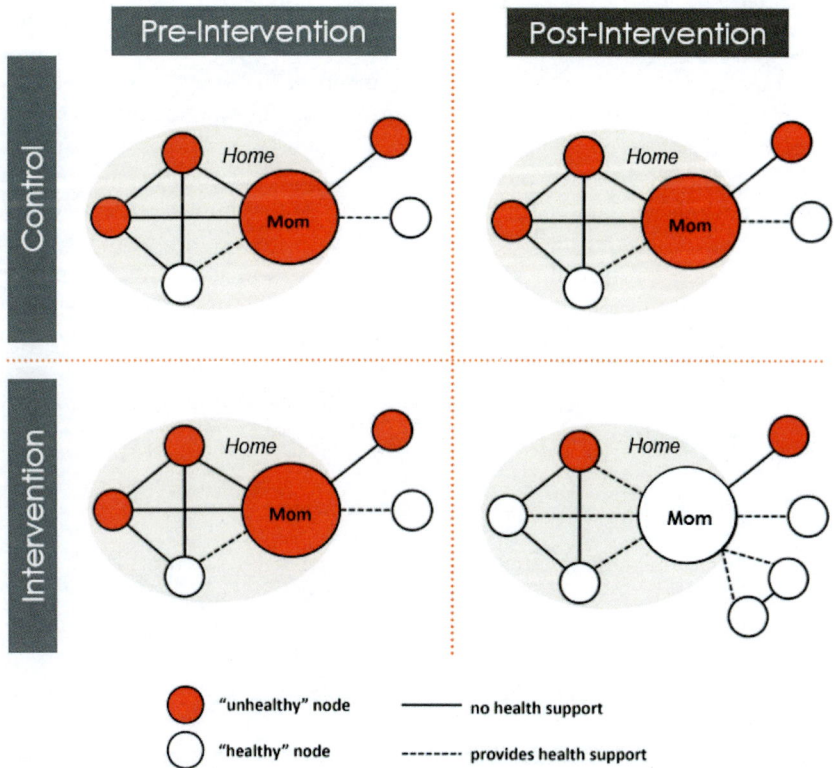

**FIGURE 3-4** Pre- and postintervention comparison of the control and intervention groups in the Healthy Home, Healthy Habits intervention.
SOURCE: Presented by Kayla de la Haye, June 30, 2020.

organizations that can support their families' healthy habits, de la Haye added, which rounds out the intervention's targeted social network changes. She described the overall goal of these changes as increasing social influence, social supports, and resources for healthy habits across mothers' home and community settings.

To illustrate the role of social network strategies in changing global environments, policies, and broader systems—which she said are often shaped by networks of community members, organizations, and decision makers—de la Haye described research that mapped networks of collaboration among organizations in a community coalition tasked with creating whole-of-community changes to prevent childhood obesity (McGlashan et al., 2019). The research examined the structure of these collaboration networks, she recounted, and how their actions mapped to the risk factors that were identified in a community causal loop diagram. According to de la Haye, the exercise provided insights into and diagnostics for these networks during implementation, as well as a method for studying how the structure of these multilayer networks supported or hindered whole-of-community change.

Lastly, de la Haye highlighted the promise of diverse and novel data sources for providing insights into complex social systems and how they evolve and affect obesity solutions. She cited as examples of data that are emerging as valuable population-level signals of social structures and social mixing big data that are captured on smartphones, such as human mobility metrics, and network information that is visible in social media. She cautioned that certain voices, relationships, and social phenomena are likely to be privileged or hidden in different data sources. Finally, she suggested that the most powerful insights into social networks and their future role in obesity solutions will be drawn from the strengths of community partnerships, survey and interview data, and emerging sources of big data and secondary data.

## PANEL DISCUSSION

Moderating a panel discussion following the presentations by Ford and de la Haye, Kumanyika began by asking the two speakers to comment on the direct relationship between the operation of racism and the operation of social networks and how both issues could be interrupted or restructured. In response, de la Haye explained that when researchers study the evolution and emergence of social networks, they often examine a rich set of variables that might predict the formation and maintenance of social ties and the exclusion of or discrimination against network members. Multiple features are often at play, she continued, and it is common to find that social selection and social mixing are based on race, ethnicity, and socioeconomic status (and on gender in children), even more so than on obesity status. With respect to inequities and the concentration of health risks among certain populations, she added, these factors contribute to the social clustering and allocation of resources, to the segregation of certain populations in broader social networks, and to exposures to different types of social environments.

Ford postulated that critical race theorists would suggest considering the differences or similarities between stigmatization ties to racialization and stigmatization ties to obesity. She highlighted one of her research projects that analyzed networks with respect to various forms of discrimination against substance abusers, and reported that people who had experienced discrimination were more likely to form their own social groups and network ties. This phenomenon, she explained, reinforced the potential for HIV risk among people who had experienced discrimination, and she added that findings of this research differed by the level of residential racial segregation in which those networks existed.

Kumanyika next invited Ford to discuss implications of the use of data with respect to facial recognition algorithms and their interpretation or in other ways. Ford referenced anecdotal evidence suggesting that health care vendors believe certain characteristics are associated with appointment truancy, and their integration of those characteristics into appointment scheduling algorithms results in longer wait times for patients with those characteristics. According to Ford, the types of general issues that will emerge from the use of big data, let alone the potential racial or racism-related issues, are not yet fully understood. Partnerships with communities are an important safeguard to facilitate the appropriate use of big data, she asserted, by ensuring transparency and access so that people understand what information is available and can drive and monitor the kinds of data that are collected. As an example of this point, she pointed to policing-related surveillance tools, which she said are developed and directed to point toward existing/prevalent or expected crime. She added that different types of tools would be needed to examine the causes of crime and to understand how analysis results derived from surveillance tools may be influenced by the person who is doing the surveillance. She added that racial justice advocates are asking these kinds of questions with regard to big data content and ownership.

Kumanyika next asked the two speakers to comment on whether efforts to help people avoid discrimination or exclusion, including in the methods used to analyze data in relation to racism and social networks as systems, are not really working against human tendencies (e.g., inclinations toward ethnocentrism and pecking orders). In response, de la Haye flagged this possibility as a potential intervention point, elaborating that researchers identify new intervention points as they gain understanding of social and network dynamics, such as the role of weight-based stigma and discrimination in network structuring. She added that the social network literature has increasingly used the concept of contagion to describe the spread of beliefs and behaviors through networks, which has highlighted that concept as a potential intervention point.

Ford remarked on the apparent parallels between systems thinking and CRT in terms of their aims to study a topic systematically, using various tools to uncover underlying, complex relationships. She expressed optimism about the promise of systems science approaches as applied to obesity solutions.

## AUDIENCE DISCUSSION

Following the panel discussion, Ford and de la Haye addressed workshop participants' questions about promoting breastfeeding as a strategy for preventing obesity, countering homophily to address obesity and other health concerns, measuring race as a social construct, addressing systemic bias favoring biological causes, and addressing structural racism while influencing systems.

### Promoting Breastfeeding as a Strategy for Preventing Obesity

A workshop participant asked about promoting breastfeeding as a strategy for preventing obesity and incorporating race and racism in breastfeeding interventions. In response, de la Haye commented that some interventions aimed at preventing obesity in the first few years of life have included breastfeeding as one component. *Promotoras* and other community-based partners, she explained, have delivered such interventions within family systems and provided insight into relevant family beliefs and cultural factors influencing breastfeeding. She identified as an emerging area of study how breastfeeding behaviors are influenced by different sources of information and influences within social networks. Kumanyika agreed with the importance of examining systems that may drive the historically lower rates of exclusive and long-duration breastfeeding among Black women.

### Countering Homophily to Address Obesity and Other Health Outcomes

A workshop participant asked about the desirability of proactively countering homophily in networks to address obesity and other health outcomes. In response, de la Haye said that countering homophily is an interesting intervention strategy because humans have evolved to connect with people with whom they can communicate and relate. People often seek out others who speak the same language, she elaborated, and feel a connection with others who share a similar background. She reported that, according to her research, stigma is a key force driving the homophily observed in health networks, such that people with selected characteristics (e.g., obesity) and health attributes are actively excluded from certain relationships. Interventions aimed at addressing stigma and discrimination, she argued, can help reduce this marginalization of certain individuals and their segregation into homophilous segments of a social network. Ford suggested that critical race analysis would pinpoint the inequality in the stigmatization of obesity (or other health condition) as the problem, rather than the homophily resulting from it.

## Measuring Race as a Social Construct

Ford responded to a workshop participant's question about how to measure race as a social construct in research settings. A first step, she offered, is to anchor race to a specific project to see how racism's operation is tied to, for instance, the experience people have when they are walking down the street and how others perceive them. She added that although the self-reported experience of racism is often held up as the ideal measure of race, how one's race is perceived by others would provide a better measure of the social experience of racism in that circumstance.

## Addressing Systemic Bias Favoring Biological Causes

Another workshop participant alleged a fundamental bias in favor of biomedical research, maintaining that despite evidence and recognition of social constructs such as race, people continue to espouse essentialism, according to which causes are at least partially biological rather than socially constructed. In response, Ford cited a lack of investment in studying the subjectivities that researchers bring to their work. She suggested that researchers regularly fill gaps in their results with their a priori assumptions. More study would be helpful, she argued, to reveal empirically the extent to which researchers do or do not reify biologically deterministic understandings of race. This process could be supported by Public Health Critical Race Praxis, which she reminded participants is intended to facilitate the application of critical race principles and methods to public health research approaches.

## Addressing Structural Racism While Influencing Systems

A workshop participant asked for examples of methods that organizations like the Roundtable on Obesity Solutions can use to address structural racism when attempting to influence complex systems. In response, de la

Haye suggested that such methods as social network analysis can provide insight beyond the perspective of individual experiences to highlight how phenomena like structural racism operate and structure people's experiences, exposures, and health risks. Ford emphasized the importance of calling racism by its name and discussing it openly. She encouraged examination of how researchers understand structural racism and how that understanding manifests in their work, as well as how structural racism operates in society and relationships.

Kumanyika stated that the process of calling out racism and understanding potentially counterproductive characteristics of social networks involves both people who are in positions of power and people who are not. She invited the speakers to suggest next steps for engaging those who have power and who benefit from structural racism or homophilic behavior that excludes others. Ford reminded workshop participants that race is a relational construct in that it has meaning when one is comparing racial groups and understanding how one group gains from another. She reiterated that it is important to avoid treating this disadvantage as an attribute of the minority population, and advocated instead for capturing it as one of the gains of the dominant group.

The importance of considering who conducts the research and collects and uses the data was stressed by de la Haye. She highlighted the focus of systems science approaches on teams that are multisector and multidisciplinary and involve and equally privilege views of community partners and other stakeholders. That inclusion is critical to understanding the data that are collected and privileged, she argued, and it is also key to promoting practices of data analysis and interpretation that can illuminate social phenomena and provide opportunities to address them.

## THE IMPACT OF NEIGHBORHOOD ENVIRONMENTS ON HEALTH

Ana Diez Roux, dean and the Distinguished University Professor of Epidemiology in the Dornsife School of Public Health at Drexel University, discussed the impact of environmental factors, particularly neighborhood characteristics, on health. She explained that neighborhoods are important contexts for physical and social exposures and can supplement individual-based explanations for health behaviors and outcomes. She also suggested that neighborhood differences may be important contributors to health inequities and that they have major public health and policy relevance because of the strong neighborhood segregation by race and income in U.S. society.

Diez Roux stressed that identifying causal effects of neighborhoods is complex because many factors drive neighborhood differences in health.

Examples of these factors include neighborhood features (e.g., availability of places to be physically active) and the sorting of people into neighborhoods based on individual attributes (e.g., people with lower incomes live in neighborhoods with fewer resources for physical activity). According to Diez Roux, much of the traditional empirical work on neighborhoods and health has attempted to disentangle the effects of a neighborhood's context from the effects of its residents' attributes in order to understand the impact of each, which she explained would help reveal causal effects. She argued, however, that the issue is much more complex because some people may be able to select where they live based on preferences for certain attributes (such as resources for physical activity), and some people may change their behavior in response to that of others around them. Furthermore, she added, neighborhoods themselves can change in response to residents' behaviors; for example, the presence of a high proportion of physically active residents may attract proprietors of recreational resources to locate in those neighborhoods. Ultimately, Diez Roux asserted, these processes form a system in which individuals and their environments evolve and interact over time to produce the neighborhood patterns that emerge, and she added that neighborhoods also affect each other.

In the face of this complexity, Diez Roux continued, interest abounds in applying systems science approaches, particularly agent-based modeling, to neighborhood effects research. According to Diez Roux and her colleagues, one reason these approaches are suitable for this research is their utility for better understanding the bidirectional person–environment relations that occur in neighborhoods, such as selection and endogeneity (e.g., understanding whether neighborhood physical activity levels increased because of local zoning and land use changes, or physically active people were more likely to move to the neighborhood because the changes made it more activity-friendly) (Auchincloss and Diez Roux, 2008). Other reasons for applying systems science approaches to this research, she added, are to better understand interactions among people, interactions and interrelations between physical and social environments, and spatial patterning (i.e., segregation) of individual and environmental characteristics.

Diez Roux highlighted research applying a particular systems science method, agent-based modeling, to explore drivers of income inequalities in diet in the context of residential segregation (Auchincloss et al., 2011). For background, she stated that income differences in dietary behaviors are well established as potential contributors to health disparities, and that spatial segregation of access to healthy food has also been documented (e.g., certain stores do not locate in lower-income neighborhoods). However, she said that questions remain regarding causality and policy implications.

According to Diez Roux, the model developed for this research was designed to address two questions. The first was whether spatial segregation contributes to income disparities in diet absent price or preference differentials, because, Diez Roux explained, it has been argued that neighborhoods simply offer what residents demand. The model was used to investigate whether the spatial segregation of stores was sufficient to generate income inequalities in diet, she elaborated, if price and preference differentials were eliminated. The second question that the model was used to address, she continued, was the degree to which price and preference manipulations affect disparities in dietary behaviors.

Diez Roux went on to explain that the two types of agents in the model are households and stores, which each have individual attributes and behaviors. She pointed out, for example, that people shop based on distance and prices, and stores react to the volume of shoppers. To address the first of the above questions, Diez Roux continued, the model compared income differentials in diet under various spatial segregation scenarios, assuming no differences between healthy and unhealthy foods in either price or preferences. It then compared income differentials holding spatial segregation constant but varying price and preferences. According to Diez Roux, the model tested different hypothetical segregation scenarios in which people with lower incomes were clustered with unhealthy stores or vice versa to see which scenario produced income differentials in diet comparable to real-world observations.

Diez Roux reported that the researchers identified a scenario most likely to result in people with higher incomes having healthier diets relative to people with lower incomes. In this scenario, lower-income households were clustered with unhealthy food stores and high-income households with healthy food stores. This result led the team to conclude that income differentials emerge in the presence of co-segregation of lower-income residents and unhealthy food stores (or higher-income residents and healthy food stores), even when food price and preferences are constant. The model then explored the effects of manipulating preferences, Diez Roux continued, such as convincing all residents to prefer healthy food. Even then, she reported, preferences could not overcome the spatial inequities, and the income differentials in dietary behaviors persisted. She added that when the model manipulated price to make healthy foods less expensive than unhealthy foods, lower-income households had better diet quality (e.g., preference for whole grains and fresh vegetables versus preference for energy-dense, nutrient-poor foods) compared with high-income households. Diez Roux remarked that this simulated outcome occurred because the relatively more expensive, unhealthy food stores closed in lower-income neighborhoods, which increased those neighborhoods' access to healthy foods.

Ultimately, Diez Roux said, the model simulation enabled the research team to conclude that segregation can create disparities in diet even if differences in price and preferences do not exist, and that changing preferences is not enough to eliminate those disparities. Price manipulation appears to have a stronger impact than that of preference manipulation, she noted, but price and preferences reinforce each other. She emphasized that the modeling exercise compelled the team to consider the processes through which dietary disparities arise, which helped generate ideas for new data collection (e.g., such variables as shopping behavior and store dynamics) and empirical analyses to fill research gaps.

Diez Roux summarized the benefits of modeling approaches, reiterating that they oblige researchers to develop dynamic conceptual models with which to illuminate mechanisms that generate associations rather than focusing on separate independent effects, account explicitly for the inter-relatedness of people and environments, and allow for input from various stakeholders. Modeling tools can yield insight through simulation, she added, and thought experiments can evaluate the effects of hypothetical interventions in a systems context.

Diez Roux next outlined caveats regarding modeling approaches. First, she advocated for "keeping it simple, but relevant." Second, she stressed that establishing transparent inclusion criteria for a model's elements is critical, as is producing data with which to support a model's assumptions, calibrate its parameters, and validate it. Developing and refining a model is an arduous process, she acknowledged, during which transparency and communication can be a challenge. Finally, she declared that a model's outputs reflect the degree of effort invested in creating it.

Diez Roux moved on to describe how systems science approaches prompt users to rethink their research questions. This may be the most valuable aspect of a systems science approach, she speculated, and she shared an example of transforming a relatively limited research question into a more nuanced, policy-relevant question:

*Original question:* Are neighborhood characteristics independently associated with health after accounting for individual-level socioeconomic status?

*Revised question:* To what extent (and under what conditions) could residential segregation generate, and reinforce, health disparities by race?

Diez Roux proposed that the toolkit for generating knowledge and evidence about population health includes modeling, observation, experimentation, action, and evaluation of action as methods that reinforce and feed back into each other. More complete understanding can be gained by combining these approaches, she argued, and by using them to quadrangulate across different methods.

Diez Roux closed her presentation by describing the SALURBAL (Salud Urbana en America Latina) study, which focused on urban environments in Latin America and health equity (Quistberg et al., 2018). She explained that one of the study's aims was to evaluate urbanicity–health–environment links and plausible policy impacts using systems thinking and simulation modeling methods, which included a participatory group model-building exercise. She described this method as engaging multiple stakeholders in building systems maps of a particular problem or process, informed by the stakeholders' lived experiences, professional backgrounds, and individual knowledge and experience. A group develops a causal loop diagram to illustrate the system, she continued, and uses it to identify critical factors as potential intervention targets and mechanisms; she added that these maps may also inform subsequent agent-based modeling.

Diex Roux ended her presentation with a quote from epidemiologist Raoul Stallones: "If we consider disease to be embedded in a complex network in which biologic, social, and physical factors all interact, then we are impelled to develop new models and adopt different analytic methods."

## INTERSECTION OF POLICY AND SYSTEMS SCIENCE MODELING TO EXAMINE SOCIAL DETERMINANTS OF PHYSICAL ACTIVITY AND OBESITY

Tiffany M. Powell-Wiley, Earl Stadtman tenure-track investigator at the National Institutes of Health and chief of the Social Determinants of Obesity and Cardiovascular Risk Laboratory, discussed the intersection of policy and systems science modeling in the context of social determinants of physical activity and obesity. She referenced the association of obesity and diabetes with premature mortality from cardiovascular disease in the United States, noting that non-Hispanic Black populations are disproportionately affected. Ideally, she suggested, interventions to address these disparities will target health behaviors related to obesity, promote health equity, and account for the social environment (Ceasar et al., 2020).

Powell-Wiley enumerated key components of her work on the relationship between cardiometabolic risk and neighborhood social environments, including perceptions of the environment and such factors as crime and safety. She also highlighted community engagement, a process in which communities help define their vision of health and suggest potential interventions, and review of epidemiologic studies, which help researchers determine how to extend the findings of community-engaged work. Systems science approaches such as simulation modeling help bridge the first two components, she explained, to support the development of interventions that account for the complexity of how social environments relate to obesity and other cardiovascular risk factors.

Powell-Wiley described how these components played out in her group's work with the Washington, DC, Cardiovascular Health and Obesity Collaborative, which she said is built on engaging communities through a community advisory board of multidisciplinary church and community leaders dedicated to addressing cardiovascular health. The board facilitates community engagement and provides input for the development and design of research projects, she explained, such as the collaborative's first project, the Washington, DC, Cardiovascular Health and Needs Assessment.

Powell-Wiley highlighted the assessment's use of principles of community-based participatory research, describing how researchers gathered data at community sites and used mixed methods to evaluate environmental and psychosocial factors related to cardiovascular risk and potential intervention tools. The assessment found that physical activity could serve as a target for improving cardiovascular health in the city's Wards 5, 7, and 8, Powell-Wiley reported, and showed the feasibility of using mobile health technology to develop a physical activity intervention. Results also indicated that community members perceived crime and limited safety as barriers to physical activity.

Powell-Wiley recounted that her group then reviewed epidemiologic studies in an attempt to extend the findings of the community-engaged work. After examining data on crime, safety, and change in cardiometabolic risk from the Multi-Ethnic Study of Atherosclerosis cohort, the researchers found an association between a greater decrease in safety over time and a greater increase in adiposity, but not a clear relationship between objective crime and adiposity (Powell-Wiley et al., 2017a). According to Powell-Wiley, this finding illuminated the concept of increased perceived safety as a potential target for intervention, which could both increase physical activity and account for residents' concerns about crime and safety.

Powell-Wiley next described the intervention's use of agent-based modeling to simulate intervention effects on community members. She explained that this method facilitates exploration of how individuals within the community interact with each other and with their environments, as well as how those relationships and environmental changes affect the system as a whole (Hammond, 2009; Nianogo and Onyebuchi, 2015). The simulation examined the impact of crime on physical activity and obesity among Black women from 80,000 households in Wards 5, 7, and 8, Powell-Wiley recalled, and community assessment data were used to validate the model. As an individual's propensity to exercise increased, reductions in crime that increased the accessibility of locations for physical activity were associated with a greater decrease in the prevalence of obesity, which she suggested showed the importance of multilevel approaches to reducing crime in order to increase leisure-time physical activity and reduce obesity (Powell-Wiley et al., 2017b). She offered as an example targeting crime through urban renewal policies so as to improve perceived safety in resource-limited urban communities.

Powell-Wiley observed that the term "urban renewal" often evokes such concepts as gentrification, which she said may have negative consequences for health equity. She shared the example of an urban renewal process with a health equity focus that is under way in Ward 8, highlighting its community economic development planning process, which engages both community residents and research partners (Mustafa, 2020). The researchers can advise community-driven efforts, she said, such as by conducting asset mapping to identify economic development opportunities that can meet community members' needs. Powell-Wiley added that in the future, her research group will be developing and using agent-based models to test multilevel mobile health interventions for promoting physical activity, and may also be testing how crime may limit the intervention.

Lastly, Powell-Wiley encouraged use of a health equity framework to guide the development of interventions focused on health promotion and health behavior change (Kumanyika, 2019). This framework, she explained, suggests four focus areas—increase healthy options, reduce deterrents, improve social and economic resources, and build on community capacity—to address when pursuing health equity for obesity prevention.

## PANEL AND AUDIENCE DISCUSSION

Corbie-Smith moderated a discussion with Diez Roux and Powell-Wiley following their presentations. She began by asking the two speakers how their systems science approaches can help build political will for structural changes to address obesity. Diez Roux replied that it has been noted that systems science approaches featuring modeling can help elucidate situations in which there is resistance to policy and in which the effects of policy are the opposite of what is intended, such as magnifying instead of reducing health equity. She argued that modeling can help stakeholders understand why those results occur and what changes could be made for policy to have its intended effect, adding that modeling can also help identify new leverage points for policies. According to Powell-Wiley, opportunity exists to build momentum for policy change by engaging community leaders in model building and use so they can visualize the potential results of different policy options.

Corbie-Smith then asked the two speakers questions submitted by workshop participants. Those questions addressed the impact of policing on community safety and physical activity, the study of systems of advantage in highly segregated White communities, and the use of models to examine the dynamics of structural racism.

## Impact of Policing in Communities

The speakers were first asked whether their research had examined the impact of policing versus other neighborhood development investment approaches. Powell-Wiley reported that her team has considered building a model to explore the impact of community policing in neighborhoods targeted by their research. She also replied to a follow-up question about nonpolicing strategies for increasing safety to increase physical activity by sharing that her team would like to study how community policing or even "violence interrupters" (i.e., individuals in the community who try to prevent escalations of violence) might impact physical activity and obesity.

## Study of Systems of Advantage in Highly Segregated White Communities

Next, Diez Roux responded to the question of whether systems of advantage, such as community investment, in highly segregated White communities have been compared with circumstances in communities where there may have been disinvestment or no investment. She suggested that systems science approaches are well suited to addressing this type of question because they can be used to explore the dynamics that occur and drive health differences, such as those by which the segregation of White advantaged residents results in certain businesses locating or not locating nearby. Systems thinking is critical for understanding drivers of health inequities, she maintained, and for understanding how structural racism affects health.

## Using Models to Examine Dynamics of Structural Racism

Powell-Wiley shared an example of her team's thinking about discrimination and segregation and their relationship to decision making about physical activity. The team considered how Black women may feel less comfortable engaging in physical activity if the people around them look different, she explained, or more comfortable if the people around them look similar. She suggested that this comfort level might affect physical activity preferences or the likelihood of engaging in physical activity, which are factors involved in this decision making.

Diez Roux argued that structural racism affects neighborhoods through the multifaceted ways in which it drives residential location. This phenomenon is related to historical redlining, she asserted, and to history that leads to differences in resources where people live. She suggested that the concentration of certain kinds of people in an area has consequences for the area (such as the location of businesses and the role of the police) as a result of institutional racism, which reinforces segregation and health inequities.

# 4

# Impacting Complex Systems That Can Influence Obesity

---

**Highlights from the Presentations of Individual Speakers**

- Engaged and participatory systems thinking strategies integrate systems science approaches and community-based participatory research. As the continuum of engaged and participatory systems thinking and community involvement progresses from a researcher's initial community outreach to shared leadership with community members, a gradual increase occurs in the level of community involvement, impact, trust, and communication flow. (Leah Frerichs)
- The connections between education and health generally fall into three categories: direct relationships, which are the ways in which school environments and interactions in the school setting interactions can impact student health; indirect relationships, which are the ways in which educational outcomes relate to later health outcomes; and causal influences of health on educational outcomes. (Matt Kasman)
- Humanistic systems science approaches balance skills in mathematics, computation, modeling, and algorithm development with the cultivation of appropriate mindsets, processes, and skills (such as curiosity, humility, compassion, and fusion and defusion) that can help researchers recognize their systematic biases and gain awareness of others' lived experiences. (Eric Hekler)

---

- Four strategies can be used to pursue structural, relational, and transformative change in communities: implementing whole-of-community approaches, leveraging community coalitions, sharing and shifting mental models, and integrating systems science approaches to engage communities in the process of understanding and changing systems. (Erin Hennessy)

The second session in Part II of the workshop explored how complex systems may influence obesity and considered opportunities for systems change as they relate to obesity solutions. Sara Czaja, professor of gerontology and director of the Center on Aging and Behavioral Research at Weill Cornell Medicine and emeritus professor of psychiatry and behavioral sciences at the University of Miami, moderated the first half of the session, during which two speakers discussed the participatory nature of interventions and education. Ihuoma Eneli, professor of clinical pediatrics at The Ohio State University, moderated the second half of the session, during which two additional speakers discussed obesity-related opportunities for systems change.

## ENGAGED AND PARTICIPATORY SYSTEMS THINKING

Leah Frerichs, assistant professor in the Department of Health Policy and Management at the University of North Carolina at Chapel Hill, discussed engaged and participatory systems thinking. She began by explaining the rationale for combining engaged and participatory research with systems thinking and systems science approaches. Synergies exist between the two, she pointed out, elaborating that both are rooted in seeking more holistic, less reductionist understanding; both emphasize socioecological frameworks and invite consideration of multilevel influences; both feature an inherent desire for capacity building and co-learning; and both involve translational synergy (Frerichs et al., 2016).

Combining the two approaches can take a variety of forms, Frerichs suggested, highlighting structured facilitated exercises—such as group model building, a systems science approach—that are designed to generate better understanding and decision making in the context of complex systems. She explained that the processes of engaged and participatory systems thinking and community engagement both reflect increasing levels of community involvement, impact, trust, and communication flow as they move through the stages of outreach, consultation, involvement, collaboration, and ultimately shared leadership. In the outreach stage, she elaborated, the researcher retains most of the power, but may conduct formative research with stakeholders to shape and refine plans. As a project moves through the later stages, she continued, researchers and community members become more equitable partners as they work together to define the issues and develop models, and perhaps even create new processes to build each other's capacity for systems thinking and action.

Frerichs then described two projects that exemplify the combining of engaged and participatory research with systems science approaches. She first displayed process flow diagrams that resulted from engaging health care providers from several community health centers in systems science work focused on processes for colorectal cancer screening. The resulting diagrams help identify health-related decision points, responsible parties for various processes, and potential gaps or bottlenecks. The formative research that led to the diagrams also informed a microsimulation model, Frerichs continued, that has been used to answer questions about the potential impact of changes in health insurance coverage on reducing the incidence of colorectal cancer and screening disparities, as well as to identify evidence-based, cost-effective interventions that can advance those goals (Davis et al., 2019; Powell et al., 2020).

Frerichs' second example was an effort to engage youth with systems science approaches in research focused on understanding complex system influences on physical activity. She described her research team's use of a shared leadership approach in working with high school students, self-titled the Young Visionaries for Health, in a rural eastern North Carolina community. The students helped the team formulate research questions and establish study protocols at the project's outset, she elaborated, and took gradually increasing responsibility for planning meetings and facilitating activities.

Frerichs explained how the project leveraged storytelling concepts to make its systems modeling components more relatable for the students. The researchers linked five storytelling elements with agent-based modeling concepts, starting by comparing conflict to the health issue (i.e., physical activity). Through simple exercises, the youth helped the researchers understand their perspectives on barriers to and supports for physical activity. Characters were equated with agents, Frerichs continued, and character development was equated with aspects of the properties and rules in the model that guided decision making. For this exercise, the students interviewed each other to elicit information about factors influencing their decisions around physical activity. The story's setting was equated with the environment; students mapped their daily routines and activity hubs on large maps of their community. Frerichs explained that the fifth element, plot, represented how the simulation played out over time. The five storytelling elements and their associated qualitative exercises contributed to the final model structure, Frerichs said, which was supplemented by youth-collected data on activities, social interactions, and locations over time. She reported that the model will soon be used to forecast the relative impact of different solutions for increasing physical activity among youth.

Concerning future directions, Frerichs expressed hope in strategies for enabling engaged systems thinking to focus on deeper, higher-impact leverage points. Referencing a continuum of increasingly greater leverage points in a system (see Figure 4-1), she remarked that leverage points at the farther end of that continuum have strong potential to create sustainable change and better address inequities relative to those at the lower end.

## A SYSTEMS SCIENCE APPROACH TO EDUCATION AND HEALTH

Matt Kasman, assistant research director at the Brookings Institution Center on Social Dynamics and Policy, discussed the use of systems science approaches to explore links between education and health. He began by highlighting two prominent efforts that situate obesity in the context of broader systems of social life: the UK Foresight Group's obesity systems map depicting the web of interconnected causal factors that affect the prevalence of obesity (see Figure 2-1 in Chapter 2), and the Lancet Commission's depiction of the global syndemic of obesity, undernutrition, and climate change, which describes how influences at multiple levels and scales link these health and ecological outcomes (see Figure 4-2). Kasman narrowed his focus within the broader systems in these figures to the connections between education and health. He offered three categories into

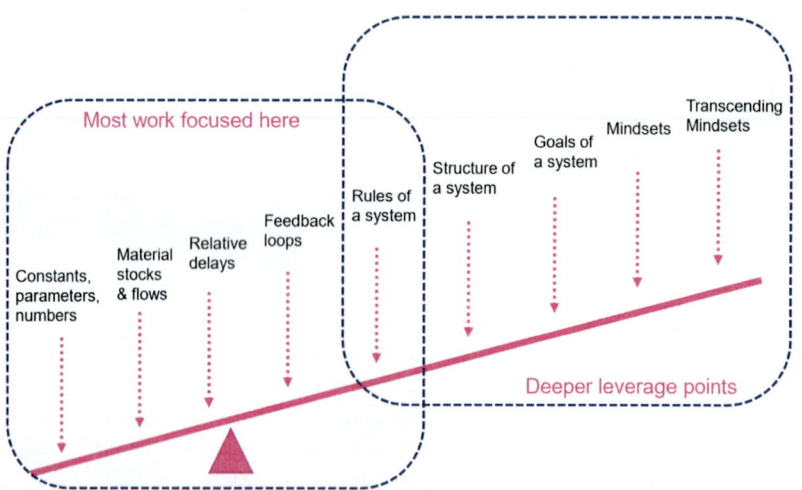

**FIGURE 4-1** Continuum of leverage points in a system.
SOURCES: Presented by Leah Frerichs, June 30, 2020 (data from Meadows, 1999). Reprinted with permission.

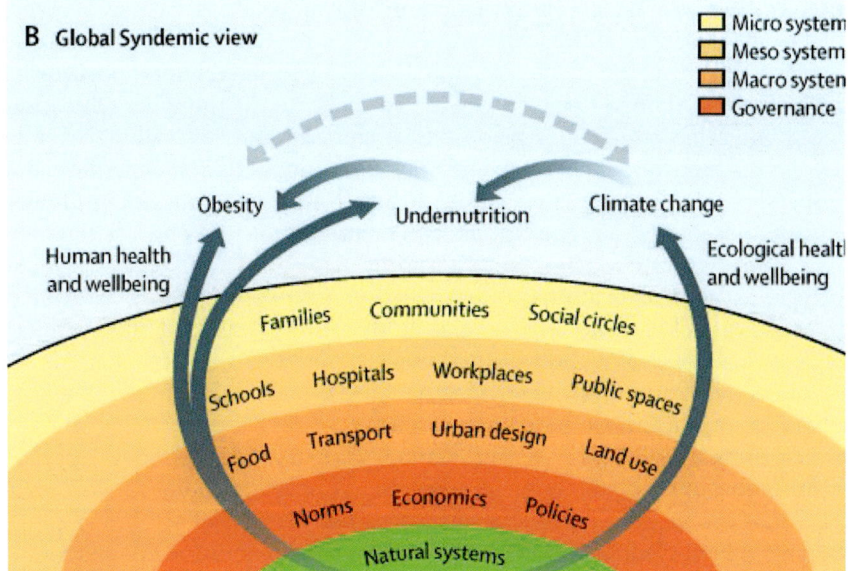

FIGURE 4-2 The global syndemic of obesity, undernutrition, and climate change.
SOURCES: Presented by Matt Kasman, June 30, 2020. Swinburn et al., 2019. Reprinted with permission.

which these connections can be placed and shared examples of systems science approaches in each category.

Kasman explained that the first category, direct relationships, includes the ways in which school environments and interactions in the school setting can impact student health, such as through access to healthy school meals and appropriate physical activity options. During the past decade or two, he remarked, many health-related systems science approaches have focused on or incorporated direct educational influences. He highlighted the National Institutes of Health (NIH)-funded COMPACT (Childhood Obesity Modeling for Prevention and Community Transformation) collaboration as a recent example, explaining that one of the key insights gained from that project is how community members from different settings, including educational institutions, can work together to effect meaningful changes that result in substantial and sustainable prevention of childhood obesity within their communities (Kasman et al., 2019; Korn et al., 2018). He suggested that COMPACT could be extended and emulated elsewhere to explore other influences on additional health outcomes.

Kasman then turned to the second category, indirect connections, or the ways in which educational outcomes relate to later health outcomes. As an example, he referenced a strong, consistent body of evidence indicating that college attendance and completion can influence later employment, place of residence, and social connections, which in turn can have important health implications. He noted that much uncertainty exists with regard to how policies and programs can make access to higher education more equitable and reduce persistent attendance gaps overall, as well as at selected institutions, by race and socioeconomic status. He mentioned a research project that created an agent-based model of college enrollment to ask and answer such questions, commenting that it is one of relatively few efforts to use systems science approaches to disentangle the myriad determinants of educational outcomes (Reardon et al., 2018). He noted the considerable potential to expand on this project and undertake similar efforts to explore other educational outcomes and treatments.

Kasman continued by describing the third category, the causal influences of health on educational outcomes, as a nascent area for research. Because of the clear linkages between education and health, he explained, causal mechanisms in the opposite direction may represent important feedback loops that operate over the long term. He suggested that these feedback loops could be critical intervention points for improving population health outcomes and reducing disparities, adding that systems science approaches could help illuminate key dynamics, disentangle interconnected causal mechanisms, and identify promising policies and interventions to promote improved outcomes.

Kasman ended his presentation by suggesting three actions to facilitate the use of systems science approaches to help understand the complex, dynamic relationships among health, educational activities, and outcomes. The first is to advocate for and use appropriate, high-quality systems science approaches to explore education and public health connections, which he said could help build familiarity with and enthusiasm for such work. The second is to increase capacity for systems science approaches, such as by developing courses and promoting mentoring relationships between experienced and new researchers. Third, Kasman urged the development of a strong community of systems science modelers, researchers, policy makers, intervention experts, and practitioners who can share inputs and expertise from a variety of backgrounds.

## PANEL DISCUSSION

Czaja moderated a panel discussion with the two speakers following their presentations. She began by asking Frerichs how the integration of engaged and participatory research with systems science approaches can be tailored for different audiences. Frerichs provided three suggestions for adapting this integrated approach. The first is to use the project's goals and research questions as guideposts, she said, and adapt them as needed when thinking about how the project activities will pursue those goals. Second, she pointed to bringing in additional critical theories and frameworks as lenses through which to view project activities and consider potential adaptations. Third, she advocated for early, equitable involvement of stakeholders in the development of project activities. Referring to the youth project she had described earlier, she mentioned experiencing tension related to overcoming the researchers' influence, explaining that it took time and flexibility to elevate the youth voices and reject the biases she had regarding the relative importance of the contributions of the researchers and youth going into the project.

Czaja next asked Kasman to offer an explanation for the lag in the uptake of the use of systems science approaches to disentangle the relationships between education and health. Kasman pointed to what he called a supply and demand issue. He described the supply as the creation of opportunities to convene experts from multiple disciplines such as education, public health, and systems science approaches. He admitted that it is a challenge to convene the right combination of people, generate a productive discussion of potential systems science approaches, and then implement a specific method. With regard to demand, Kasman postulated that funders, large research organizations, publication venues, and policy makers will have heightened interest in systems science approaches as they become aware of the power and potential of those approaches to aid in examining complex issues. As these approaches reveal important linkages between education and health, he submitted, the demand for additional systems science research will grow.

Kasman also argued for the importance of both formal and informal means of collaboration and encouraged involving educators and students in systems thinking. As an example of cross-sector collaboration, he shared that school administrators and educators in San Francisco were willing to collaborate with him on his doctoral dissertation examining the relationships of school choice and student assignment policies with levels of racial segregation in schools. The education stakeholders provided valuable data and helped shape the research questions, he explained, noting that had his research involved a public health question, he would have needed to involve public health stakeholders to provide another layer of buy-in, content expertise, and data.

Finally, Czaja asked the two speakers for thoughts on integrating their approaches. Kasman suggested that the participatory nature of Frerichs' approach could help elicit valuable research questions and insights for integration in a simulation model, and that data from single settings could be generalized to suggest what might work to achieve similar outcomes in different contexts. Frerichs echoed the notion that important linkages could be made between education and health, recalling that educational factors, such as emotional stressors of school, have been raised in her work to support physical activity among youth.

## AUDIENCE DISCUSSION

Following their panel discussion, Frerichs and Kasman answered workshop participants' questions about engaging stakeholders in systems science approaches, cultivating diverse skill sets to succeed with those approaches, and addressing the potential for disparities due to virtual schooling and physical activity programs.

### Engaging Stakeholders in Systems Science Approaches

Frerichs highlighted scripts for group model building, such as Scriptapedia,[1] in response to a request for resources with which to engage stakeholders in systems science approaches. She also mentioned the Creative Learning Exchange,[2] which aims to develop "systems citizens" in K–12 education, pointing to the potential use of its resources for engaging stakeholders in the education system. Kasman suggested engaging audiences by showing them the results of systems science approaches, such as dynamic visualizations. He highlighted two examples of these products: a resource focused on the effect of college subsidies on recipients' enrollment,[3] and the Tobacco Town modeling (see the summary of Douglas Luke's presentation in Chapter 2). According to Kasman, these resources help stakeholders answer questions about which policies might work for their specific contexts, and then disseminate that information in a vivid way to generate enthusiasm.

### Cultivating Diverse Skill Sets to Succeed with Systems Science Approaches

A workshop participant commented on the emerging challenge of an implied need for systems science researchers to have a range of skills, such as robust mathematics and computation abilities, as well as strengths in understanding people, including themselves. These are classically siloed skill sets, Czaja pointed out, and she asked Frerichs and Kasman to suggest solutions for overcoming unintended consequences of classic disciplinary boundaries. Frerichs voiced her own challenges with striving to build skills in multiple areas, and suggested the strategies of creating multidisciplinary teams and working with youth to build a pipeline of systems thinkers.

---

[1] See https://en.wikibooks.org/wiki/Scriptapedia (accessed October 9, 2020).
[2] See www.clexchange.org (accessed September 17, 2020).
[3] See www.brookings.edu/interactives/education-subsidies-code (accessed September 17, 2020).

Kasman stated that education and public health are areas in which traditional boundaries between quantitative and qualitative work are breaking down in a good way. He pointed to a growing understanding of the importance of using qualitative findings to build a sense of external validity and an intuition about how causal mechanisms operate, as well as a recognition of how quantitative methodologies can help identify tipping points and time scales.

### Addressing the Potential for Disparities Due to Virtual Schooling and Physical Activity Programs

A workshop participant asked whether virtual fitness programs to encourage movement regardless of location or social or cultural background are an effective way to help the most vulnerable people. Frerichs related the question to the relationship between social distancing and health, saying that her work with youth has revealed the importance of social connections to being healthy and active. Kasman urged remaining alert to unintended consequences of virtual programs that could exacerbate existing disparities, referencing emerging evidence of a growing divide in educational progress and academic achievement due to widespread remote schooling amid the coronavirus disease 2019 (COVID-19) pandemic. Uninterrupted access to virtual learning supports is unevenly distributed among the population, he explained, and he advocated for more equitable access to resources and user supports. He pointed out as well that equitable access to virtual physical activity resources is an important aspect of preventing a worsening of disparities in that realm.

Czaja asked the speakers which factors contribute to remote schooling–induced disparities in educational outcomes. Kasman stressed that empirical evidence of such disparities is only now emerging, but suggested that they result from a confluence of factors. He mentioned in particular the reliability of Internet access, the conduciveness of the residential setting to learning (e.g., noise level, interruptions), and access to technology and user support for that technology. Frerichs agreed and appealed for approaching issues from an asset-based approach focused on leveraging community resilience and other strengths.

### HUMANISTIC SYSTEMS SCIENCE TO FOSTER BEHAVIOR CHANGE

Eric Hekler, director of the Center for Wireless & Population Health Systems and associate professor in the Department of Family Medicine & Public Health at the University of California, San Diego, spoke about using systems science approaches to foster behavior change. Before starting his presentation, he noted that the university resides on the unceded territory of the Kumeyaay Nation.

Hekler recalled a quote from Albert Einstein, "as simple as possible, but not simpler," as he recounted the moment when he recognized the tremendous mismatch between the complexity of trying to help people live healthy lives and the randomized controlled trials being applied to the problem. He outlined three dimensions to consider with regard to behavior change: the importance of contextual factors, the dynamic nature of those factors, and the idiosyncratic nature of how different factors influence an individual. The complexity of these dimensions calls for solutions that are as simple as possible, he argued, but not simpler.

Heckler then turned to three lessons from his evolving thinking about advancing systems science approaches to match the complexity of human behavior change. First, he espoused a focus on verbs (i.e., dynamics, interconnectivity, and flows within and across systems) instead of nouns (i.e., interventions, levels, and outcomes). He elaborated on this lesson by giving an overview of control systems engineering, which he described as a large, pervasive field focused on dynamic decision making in complex environments. Control systems focus on the dynamics of each individual system involved in a process, he explained, and he gave the example of the role of a health coach as a control system for weight management. A health coach represents a theoretical model of health behavior change, he elaborated, and selects from a variety of tools to promote that change, such as goal setting or reward programs. Health coaches also have tools to help people monitor their activities, he noted, and can make adjustments based on how people respond.

Control systems use a technique called system identification to build dynamic models based on data from an actual person or other unit of interest, Hekler continued, and the models feed into simulations of how the person will respond in future scenarios. He used as an example that stress prompts some people to walk more and others to walk less, a difference that can be incorporated into a model. Because models specify decision points mathematically, he explained, they can account for changing contexts and honor interpersonal differences as they determine the best decisions over a specified timeline in order to reach a goal.

Hekler cautioned that an unintended consequence of building control algorithms is that they can manipulate people, a recognition that he said led him to his second lesson: whoever defines success and categories has the power. Such decisions are better left to the people being served by systems science tools, he maintained, and he urged opening innovation pathways for nontraditional researchers and experts to contribute to these tools. As an example, he described how a nonengineering colleague with type 1 diabetes working outside of her discipline was able to build and distribute the plans for an artificial pancreas system.

The third lesson, Hekler continued, is the importance of humanistic systems science training, which combines training in mathematics, computation, modeling, and algorithm development with the cultivation of humanistic scientists characterized by appropriate mindsets, processes, and interpersonal skills. Noting that scientists tend to have systematic biases and privileges, he shared his personal experience with overcoming what he called "confident ignorance and emotional blindness." Recalling situations in which he stepped back and allowed nontraditional partners to drive efforts, he said the result was greater capacity to build equitable participation. Hekler espoused the qualities of curiosity, humility, and compassion as key ingredients for recognizing one's biases and building awareness of others' lived experiences. He urged attention to the processes of triangulation, study of root causes, and iteration, and advocated for building skills in fusion and defusion, listening, and synthesizing.

Another facet of the third lesson, Hekler continued, is that humanistic systems science would benefit from acting more like a GPS and less like a yardstick. The latter approach specifies an end goal, he explained, but dynamic systems are constantly managing inputs that warrant different goals based on the context. He urged that behavior change processes be attuned to context to determine what outcomes are most desirable under different circumstances (Schraefel and Hekler, 2020).

## OBESITY-RELATED OPPORTUNITIES FOR SYSTEMS CHANGE IN COMMUNITIES

Erin Hennessy, assistant professor in the Friedman School of Nutrition Science and Policy at Tufts University, discussed the use of systems thinking and systems science approaches to advance community-level obesity prevention. An iceberg model is often used to explain systems thinking and systems change, Hennessy began, because it is an apt illustration of how a visible outcome, such as obesity, is the manifestation of an underlying collection of factors that lie below the surface (see Figure 4-3). She explained that these factors include trends (e.g., poor diet and inactivity), structures (e.g., policies, practices, resource flows), and relational aspects (relationships and connections, power dynamics) that drive obesity-related trends and events, as well as mental models, which she described as deeply held beliefs, assumptions, and operating styles that influence one's thoughts, speech, and actions (Kania et al., 2018).

Hennessy noted that the structural, relational, and mental model elements exist with varying degrees of visibility to players in the system, yet typically play a significant role in such problems as obesity. Therefore, she argued, they are promising leverage points for effecting systems change. Although the less explicit factors (such as relationships and connections,

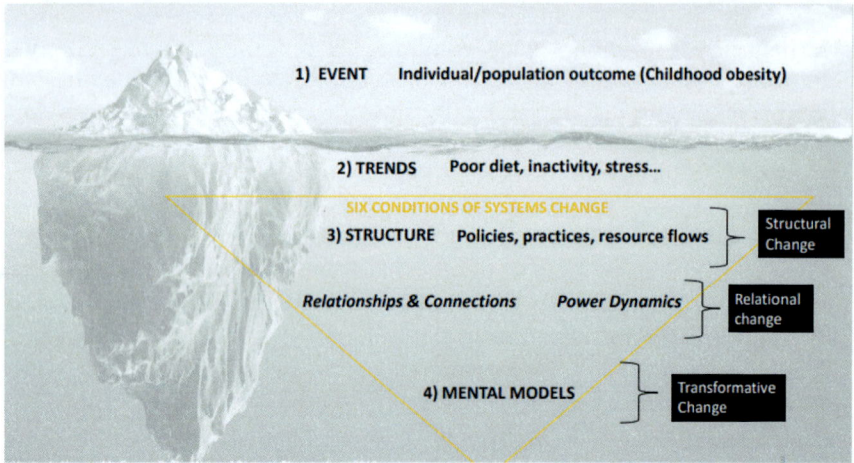

**FIGURE 4-3** Iceberg model illustrating systems thinking and systems changes.
SOURCES: Presented by Erin Hennessy, June 30, 2020 (data from Kania et al., 2018).
Reprinted with permission.

power dynamics, and mental models) are challenging to clarify, she maintained that their tremendous potential to shift a system warrants their consideration in efforts to effect change.

Hennessy next turned to discussing the promise of whole-of-community approaches for effecting systems changes to prevent obesity. These approaches are multilevel, multifaceted, and implemented holistically throughout an entire community, she explained, and target multiple levels of influence and behaviors through policy, practice, and resource flows. They have the potential to be effective and equitable when focused on structural components, she added, as well as when intervention strategies target a variety of contexts and when the community is engaged.

Hennessy cited community engagement as a key element of a second opportunity for systems changes to prevent obesity—leveraging community coalitions, which she described as groups of leaders and stakeholders from diverse organizations, settings, and sectors working collectively on a common objective within the local context, perhaps even within a whole-of-community approach. This combination is particularly promising, Hennessy asserted, because coalition members can devote energy and resources to implementing structural changes and share critical information and resources specific to local contexts. Furthermore, she noted, coalitions have been observed to collaborate, build relationships and community capacity, and plan and diffuse tailored interventions (Korn et al., 2018).

Hennessy described the Shape Up Somerville study as an example of a community-wide intervention that leveraged a community-based participatory research approach to make structural and relational changes to prevent obesity. She explained that the intervention's policy and environmental changes were designed and diffused through a community coalition, the Shape Up Somerville Taskforce, and resulted in a significant decrease in body mass index (BMI) z-scores among children living in an intervention community (Hennessy et al., 2020). She then displayed a systems map of Somerville's dynamics of community change, which she described as a qualitative systems modeling approach to visualizing the entire system's interactions and success factors. She flagged the map's inclusion of the stakeholders' mental models with regard to underlying processes that drove the adoption, dissemination, implementation, and sustainability of the intervention (Hennessy et al., 2020).

Hennessy reported that the Shape Up Somerville systems map also alerted the investigators to the role of the Shape Up Taskforce in the intervention's success (Hennessy et al., 2020). This realization helped articulate a new theory called stakeholder-driven community diffusion, she explained, which posits that community coalitions drive successful interventions by leveraging social network structures to diffuse their knowledge and engagement with the public health prevention effort across the broader community. That diffusion creates community readiness to implement and sustain change, Hennessy added, and mobilizes change agents who can catalyze bottom-up demand. She noted that efforts are under way to generate empirical evidence on the contributions of coalitions to whole-of-community interventions for improving childhood obesity outcomes.

Hennessy moved on to share a third opportunity for systems change at the community level: sharing and shifting mental models. Mental models inform decision-making processes, she stated, but if those models are not explicit, stakeholders may harbor different perspectives and beliefs about a problem and develop disparate, siloed solutions. Systems science approaches such as community-based system dynamics (CBSD) provide a method for involving communities in the process of understanding and changing systems. Hennessy explained that CBSD is a means of community capacity building and a technique for equalizing power among group members, enabling input from all participants and promoting group cohesion. She cited group model building as another approach for involving stakeholders in the modeling process, in which trained facilitators follow scripted group exercises to lead diverse stakeholders through a process of defining and eventually visualizing a complex and dynamic system, allowing them to develop and prioritize action steps and build connections across time and scale (Calancie et al., 2020).

Hennessy identified integrating systems science approaches as a fourth opportunity for community-level systems change, enabling expansion of the research questions that can be asked and yielding novel insights. She described her team's use of multiple approaches to help understand the mechanisms by which community coalitions diffuse evidence-based interventions in a community (Hennessy et al., 2020). The team used systems mapping to generate an initial hypothesis, she recounted, then expanded that hypothesis to a full mechanistic theory that was tested with agent-based modeling.

Community-based system dynamics and group model building have been employed as intervention strategies, Hennessy continued, to guide multisector community coalitions through a process of extracting mental models, building collective understanding of a complex problem, and committing to actions to address the problem. She explained that her team's agent-based model defines agents as community coalition stakeholders who possess knowledge, engagement, and position in a social network, which Hennessy said allows for a quantitative, computational strategy for understanding longitudinal change in these key metrics. She added that social network analysis is used to measure and test diffusion of the coalition's knowledge and engagement.

In closing, Hennessy circled back to the iceberg model to reiterate how different systems science approaches facilitate a focus on the underlying elements that influence systems change (e.g., using social network analysis to study relational elements or group model building to explore mental models).

## PANEL DISCUSSION

Eneli moderated a panel discussion with Hekler and Hennessy following their presentations, starting with a question about how and with whom power dynamics manifest within systems. She also asked for examples of systems science approaches that have been useful for addressing health equity in communities.

Hennessy referenced her training in community-based participatory research, which she said involves a perspective that all parties have expertise to contribute to addressing a complex problem such as obesity. She mentioned community-based system dynamics and group model building as systems science methods that her team has used with community coalitions across the United States, adding that researchers have had to be cognizant of their own biases to ensure that they are building sustainable capacity for the community to continue the work when researchers leave. She explained that researchers train coalition organizers and leaders in these methods and provide ongoing support so they can use the methods over time. She added that although these two methods help equalize power dynamics, tension exists as participants question each other's inclusion in the process, the goals of the process, and what evidence-based strategies will be implemented.

Hekler cautioned that collective action can do harm even with the best intentions because people often do not realize the connections between generalization and colonization as constructs or recognize that micro-aggressions matter. He suggested that people could begin to recognize deep systemic issues by learning lessons from history, sociology, anthropology, and economics that focus on inequities. He suggested that building a safe space for others to provide feedback helps prevent people from propagating what he had referred to in his presentation as "confident ignorance," and that such two-way conversations can be achieved by building safety and trust among participants. Referencing speakers who had reflected on their experiences that have imparted lessons for building humility, Hekler advocated for a commitment to values and virtues, as well as for building sufficient but not excess confidence in oneself so as to feel secure in conversations and have productive discussions.

## AUDIENCE DISCUSSION

Next, Hekler and Hennessy responded to workshop participants' questions about immutable versus evolving factors in systems, similarities and differences across communities as observed in experiences with community-engaged efforts to address obesity, and fusion and defusion skills.

### Immutable Versus Evolving Factors in Systems

In response to a question about how researchers applying systems science approaches handle immutable factors, Hekler confirmed that some factors truly cannot be changed, but urged careful thought about the distinction between truly immutable and evolving factors. He suggested that some factors may appear immutable, but in reality are changing on a time scale that is slower than what the human mind typically encounters. He reiterated the importance of examining the dynamics of how factors are moving and changing. Hennessy concurred that tension exists in this area, noting that some systems models have been used to explore factors that have been framed by some researchers as nonmodifiable and by others as modifiable. She reiterated that combinations of systems science approaches are needed to tackle complex problems such as obesity.

### Similarities and Differences Across Communities

Hennessy addressed a question about lessons learned from her work on the Shape Up Somerville initiative, stating that although no two communities are alike, sufficient similarities may exist across the contextual factors, practices, and policies that sustain obesity to produce a high-level framework to guide the work of community coalitions like the Shape Up Somerville Taskforce. One aspect of such a framework, she noted, is to suggest which sectors and stakeholders are important to include in community coalitions. She also pointed to one similarity across communities—the ability to do powerful, dynamic work without substantial financial resources, instead leveraging relationships and resource flows to diffuse evidence-based interventions—while acknowledging that different contextual factors, such as political dynamics, certainly exist, and communities sometimes conceptualize problems differently.

### Fusion and Defusion Skills

Another workshop participant asked Hekler to elaborate on his suggestion that scientists cultivate the skills of fusion and defusion. Hekler explained that the general concept involves cultivating the ability to fuse or defuse with one's experiences. An example of fusing with one's experience would be to say, "I am angry," he said, whereas defusing the experience on multiple levels might look like saying, "I am having the experience of anger with others in my home." The latter, higher-level perspective, he explained, allows people to see themselves as part of a system. He added that fusion is appropriate in certain situations, such as when trying to see oneself as part of a community or striving to be emotionally present with others, whereas other situations call for defusion, such as when examining the systemic biases that one may bring to a project. These skills go beyond simply trying to be objective, he maintained.

# 5

# Examples from the Field: Applying Systems Thinking to Population Health Issues

---

**Highlights from the Presentations of Individual Speakers**

- A key strategy for promoting a more physically active lifestyle is to make physical activity accessible for people at different levels of fitness and self-efficacy, such as by providing relatable models and a variety of activity options to suit a range of fitness levels. (John Jakicic)
- Multilevel interventions to treat obesity produce larger and longer-lasting effects relative to interventions that target only one level of the socioecological model. It is important to understand multilevel systems synergies and constraints on implementing an obesity intervention, and to continually optimize such interventions for both effectiveness and efficiency. (Bonnie Spring)
- Causal loop diagrams help community stakeholders see where they fit into a response to obesity and can be used to track actions and visualize actors, actions, and the connections among them. Researchers can better understand the complexities of childhood obesity by using a range of systems science approaches, combining methods, and collaborating. (Steve Allender)

---

The workshop's final session featured three speakers who shared field examples of how research is exploring the application of systems thinking to address obesity and population health. Sara Bleich, professor of public health policy at the Harvard T.H. Chan School of Public Health and the Carol K. Pforzheimer Professor in the Radcliffe Institute for Advanced Study at Harvard University, moderated the session.

## PHYSICAL ACTIVITY

John Jakicic, director of the Healthy Lifestyle Institute and chair of the Department of Health and Physical Activity at the University of Pittsburgh, discussed examples of integrating systems and sectors to promote physical activity. He described his university's work as a "living laboratory" that aims to translate research center–based initiatives into broader, institution- and community-based initiatives. He expounded on lessons learned from the process of translating initiatives into these broader systems contexts.

The research center–based initiatives, Jakicic began, revolve around physical activity for the prevention and treatment of obesity. They involve classical measurements collected in controlled laboratory settings, randomization, and participant eligibility criteria, he said, and they provide signals of things that could work in the field even though they do not fully represent real-world settings.

Jakicic explained that laboratory work in research settings helps form a foundation for the content that is applied in institution-based initiatives. He shared examples of his team's translation of learnings from the research environment into interventions within the broader University of Pittsburgh setting, which employs 15,000 adults. The team believed that building a community of physical activity in the university environment was a precursor to expanding that community beyond the university setting, he noted, and then throughout the city of Pittsburgh more broadly.

Jakicic reported that the team began by surveying members of the university community about supports for physical activity, and received feedback centered on a desire for more exercise facilities and equipment. He pointed out, however, that targeting exercise is markedly different from promoting physical activity. Furthermore, he continued, the team determined that only a small percentage of adults at the university (estimated by Jakicic as approximately 500 out of 15,000 people) are regular fitness center users; therefore, an investment in additional facilities and equipment would likely not reach the vast majority of the target audience. Jakicic also described feedback from individuals not engaged in exercise who indicated that they avoided fitness facilities for such reasons as intimidation (i.e., the perception that their relative lack of knowledge about how to engage in structured exercise would make them feel out of place), dislike of their appearance when they exercised, and dislike of exercise in general. However, he said, these individuals were willing to engage in other forms of physical activity.

The survey findings, Jakicic continued, led the team to think more broadly about the kinds of initiatives that would draw the rest of the university population into a more physically active lifestyle. He described his team's discovery that a key element of building a community of physical activity is to make people feel as though they are part of something together with others who are just like them. This discovery, he said, led to the birth of the Be Fit Pitt initiative, which attracted people who were not regular exercisers but who wished to move more as they viewed activity from the perspective of a healthier lifestyle. The team drew on laboratory research–based findings indicating that individuals with low activity levels are more likely to sustain physical activity if new activity options are introduced every 8 to 12 weeks, which prompted the creation of regular programming opportunities for engagement in physical activity. Jakicic mentioned several themed activities that leveraged holidays, encouraged friendly competition, and engaged people in fun ways to be active. The initiative started to catch on, he recounted, and grew as the university community was creatively activated on an ongoing basis and activities were modified over time.

Gradually, Jakicic continued, the team introduced remote opportunities for people to engage in physical activity, such as livestreamed or recorded video activities. The benefit of this strategy, he explained, is that it satisfies participants' desire to engage in physical activity without feeling the intimidation of being visible. He highlighted PittWire Live as an example of an online platform that has received positive feedback, explaining that its livestreamed physical activity sessions are able to reach communities beyond the university campus.

Jakicic went on to describe how his team approached expanding the Be Fit Pitt initiative into the broader community. They quickly learned that the traditional exercise facilities in communities were often small, dingy, and generally unappealing, he reported, which propelled them to consider more engaging ways to activate people. He described how they discovered that a key strategy was to make activity accessible for people at different levels of fitness and self-efficacy, such as by providing relatable models and a variety of activity options to suit people's varying fitness levels. Jakicic acknowledged, however, that livestreamed programming does not work for communities without adequate computer equipment and reliable Internet access, and he urged initiatives to consider how to reach the largest possible number of people.

Finally, Jakicic highlighted examples of how the University of Pittsburgh partners with surrounding communities to understand what would work to encourage and facilitate physical activity in their unique contexts. He described community engagement centers, where university representatives host community discussions not for the purpose of formal research, but to understand community needs and assets.

## DESIGN OF MULTILEVEL INTERVENTIONS FOR OBESITY

Bonnie Spring, professor of preventive medicine, psychology, psychiatry, and public health at Northwestern University and director of its Center for Behavior and Health within the Institute for Public Health and Medicine, discussed the design of multilevel interventions to treat obesity. She began by describing a basic premise of the socioecological intervention framework: interventions that target determinants at multiple levels of that framework produce larger and longer-lasting effects relative to interventions that target only one level (Weiner et al., 2012). With regard to clinical treatment of obesity, Spring pointed to the Diabetes Prevention Program (DPP), which the U.S. Preventive Services Task Force considers the "gold standard." She described the DPP as an intensive, multicomponent behavioral treatment, which grew out of a successful weight loss and diabetes prevention intervention that was tested in multiple sites in 2002. Initially, the DPP treatment package involved 24 one-on-one, in-person treatment sessions led by health professional counselors, Spring explained, but now it is common to have group sessions led by trained lay counselors at a much lower cost.

Spring described how her team optimized the DPP by studying which additional dimensions of the socioecological model beyond the individual level produced enhanced weight loss when targeted by the intervention (see Figure 5-1). She explained that all participants received a core intervention that was remote and targeted the individual level by promoting app-based self-monitoring of daily weight, dietary intake, and physical activity, as well as by providing coaching calls. Half of the participants received 12 calls from a coach who offered counseling based on the digitally transmitted self-monitoring data, while the remainder of the participants received more intensive coaching consisting of 24 calls. All participants joined the trial with a support buddy. Spring explained that the intervention targeted the interpersonal level for half of the sample by training the support buddies in how to provide support; buddies for the remainder of the sample received no such training. The intervention targeted the organizational level, Spring said, by sending weight loss progress reports to the primary care providers for half of the sample but not the remainder. She acknowledged that the environmental and policy level posed more of a challenge, but the intervention was able to offer 1 week of portion-controlled meal replacements and then recommendations for meal replacements in subsequent weeks. Ultimately, Spring said, the intervention aimed to discover which treatment components would contribute most to 6-month weight loss and at what cost.

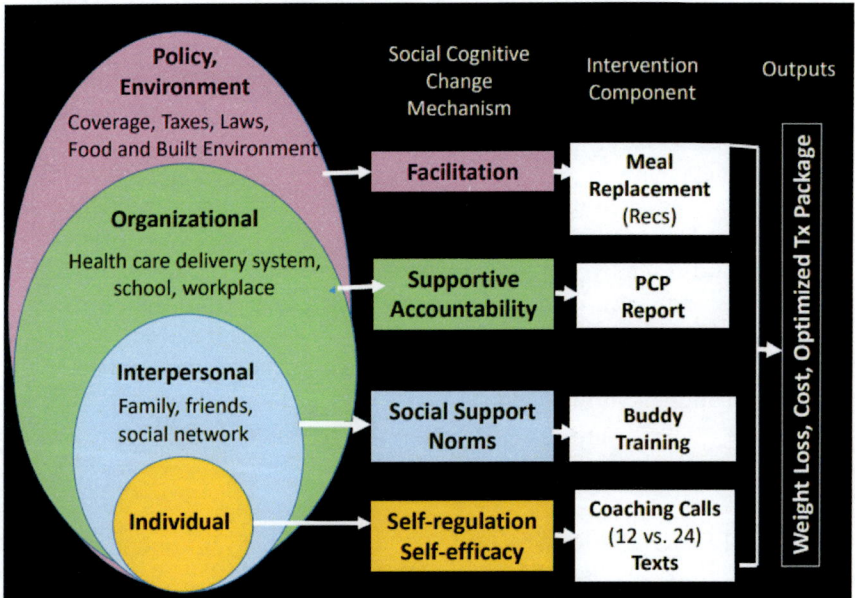

**FIGURE 5-1** Ecological model for obesity intervention.
NOTE: PCP Report = primary care provider weight loss report; Recs = recommendations; Tx = treatment.
SOURCE: Presented by Bonnie Spring, June 30, 2020. Reprinted with permission.

Turning to the intervention results, Spring noted that 562 people were randomized, and the 6-month retention rate was 84.3 percent. The component that significantly increased weight loss was buddy support, she reported, an effect that was enhanced when the weight loss progress report was sent to a primary care provider. Perhaps the reason why 24 coaching calls produced no more weight loss than 12 calls, she hypothesized, was because participants' self-regulation training needs were met by the lower level of coaching. Thus, additional weight loss was not seen unless the intervention also targeted the interpersonal and organizational levels of the ecological model. Spring reviewed a table populated with the intervention data to demonstrate how to build a treatment package that maximizes 6-month weight loss for less than $500: a remotely delivered weight loss intervention comprising an app, 12 digitally connected coaching sessions, buddy training, and primary care progress reports produced 7 percent weight loss for 52 percent of the sample, a result comparable to that of the original DPP in-person intervention at less burden and cost ($427). Particularly when limited resources call for best-value solutions to extend treatment to the greatest number of people, Spring added, a $324 trimmed-down version of the intervention involving only the app plus 12 coaching calls produced 5 percent weight loss for 53 percent of the sample (Spring et al., 2020).

Spring went on to discuss how the DPP has moved from hospital- and health care–based delivery systems into community settings. The program has been scaled successfully in YMCAs, she reported, yet engages relatively few of its intended recipients. She asserted that this is the case because place-based programs present such barriers as transportation and child care, which disenfranchises the target audience. Spring called for linkages that can promote both scale and reach by spanning the dimensions of care delivery, community services, and family and individual engagement and empowerment.

In summary, Spring maintained that multilevel interventions are promising and encouraged understanding multilevel systems synergies and constraints on implementing obesity interventions. Finally, she appealed for continual optimization for effectiveness and efficiency within the context of change.

## LESSONS FROM COMMUNITY-BASED OBESITY PREVENTION IN AUSTRALIA

Steve Allender, professor of population health and founding director of the Global Obesity Center (a World Health Organization Collaborating Center for Obesity Prevention) at Deakin University, shared lessons from community-based obesity prevention trials in Victoria, Australia. He described a relatively new and commonly used trial design, a stepped wedge cluster randomized trial in which some intervention communities are active at earlier and others at later points in the study. The trial design builds on a 20-year history of community-based interventions, which Allender said imparted several lessons: childhood obesity is preventable; community-led interventions targeting various stages of childhood can be effective; multilevel strategies are important; local ownership and leadership are critical; implementation is often time-consuming and challenging; and if these lessons are not applied, sustainability is likely to be limited, especially in a climate of fluctuation in political support. According to Allender, these lessons helped researchers recognize the importance of giving communities tools and techniques to address the complexity of conditions because their contexts are vastly different.

Allender next provided an overview of the intervention in Victoria, which follows a nonlinear process. An early step is to engage a catalyst in each community, whom he described as a person who is well-connected and motivated to do the work. Researchers work with the catalyst to engage local leadership, he explained, using methods from systems science approaches, particularly system dynamics and group model building, to develop a shared understanding of the complexity of the causes and outcomes of overweight and obesity in each community. According to Allender, the researchers' role is to provide the evidence base and help the community understand how it might inform community action, and then to support the community's momentum for change by building capacity; providing tools and resources; and providing monitoring, evaluation, and feedback.

Allender displayed a causal loop diagram constructed by community stakeholders as part of a whole-of-systems approach to addressing childhood overweight and obesity in Campbelltown, Australia. The diagram is color-coded, he explained, to distinguish subsystems of interest such as physical activity, nutrition, education, and social determinants of health. A benefit of the causal loop diagram, he observed, is that community stakeholders can begin to see where they best fit into a response to obesity. Another is that it can be used to track actions corresponding to the issues illustrated by the diagram, he added, recounting that 8 actions had been taken 3 months into the intervention and 63 actions by the 2-year mark. The actions operate at multiple levels and in different parts of the community, he pointed out, but most important, they are backed by community interest and capacity.

Next, Allender highlighted STICKE,[1] software invented by his group to help communities facilitate the process of creating causal loop diagrams and tracking actors and actions. He showed a portion of the Campbelltown causal loop diagram that included actors, actions, and the connections among them. Some of the connections represent new relationships among stakeholders, he noted, who have joined together with a new focus on specific actions to improve child health. Allender observed that tracking of actions has revealed the scope of topics that communities are addressing. He referenced a community in Western Victoria that was part of the Whole of Systems Trial of Prevention Strategies for childhood obesity (WHO STOPS childhood obesity) study, with 480 actions in some level of implementation. It was encouraging to see that many of the actions were related to healthy eating, he remarked, which aligned with evidence suggesting the need to emphasize food choices.

Sharing interim results, Allender reported that on average these community-based trials result in a 4 percent reduction in the prevalence of overweight and obesity over the first 2 years, but he noted that further work is needed to understand the longer-term outcomes. He added that significant improvement is seen in health-related quality of life among children in the intervention communities, as are positive changes in obesity-related behaviors over the long term. By combining a range of methods with systems science approaches, Allender said, researchers can better understand and respond to the complexity of childhood obesity.

---

[1] See https://sticke.deakin.edu.au (accessed October 5, 2020).

## AUDIENCE DISCUSSION

Bleich moderated a discussion with the three speakers following their remarks. The discussion covered community perceptions of systems science approaches, technology to enable remote delivery of interventions, reconciling individual perspectives with systems science approaches, engaging the private sector, and lessons from community engagement.

### Community Perceptions of Systems Science Approaches

Bleich asked Allender to describe how communities in Australia perceive a systems science approach to obesity prevention compared with a more traditional approach. Allender replied that a systems science approach is more logical from a community's point of view, and described how his team presents this approach as a way of thinking that might be helpful and then allows communities to opt in to proceed. Gaining initial buy-in from the community instills a level of confidence among community leaders, he added, who might risk a loss of social capital if they agreed to an approach disliked by community members. Group model building occurs at the beginning of the intervention, he continued, which excites the community to keep moving forward as it becomes possible to visualize the problem with its complexity and feedback loops. According to Allender, this process helps community members find ways to work together that are evidence-informed and respect the complexity of the problem and its context, a benefit that traditional methods cannot provide.

### Technology to Enable Remote Delivery of Interventions

Bleich asked Spring to suggest solutions for the challenges of recruitment and retention of participants for YMCA-based DPPs. Spring replied that potential participants are dispersed across many different geographic areas, and may have limited time and resources to attend in-person treatment sessions. She observed that the coronavirus disease 2019 (COVID-19) pandemic has illuminated the promise of delivering interventions remotely, and mentioned studies indicating positive results from delivering the DPP with online and asynchronous Internet communication via federally qualified health centers. She pointed out that people often perceive technology as a limiting factor for underresourced communities, but that what she termed a "reverse digital divide" exists for access to mobile tools. She noted that Black and Hispanic communities have used mobile health tools extensively, and suggested that these tools may be promising for outreach to older adults if they are taught how to use them and can access technological support as needed. Jakicic concurred, referencing a survey of older adults indicating that a majority want to have remote options for receiving help. He hypothesized that this finding may reflect a desire for convenience and regular touchpoints.

### Reconciling Individual Perspectives with Systems Science Approaches

Recalling the finding by Jakicic's team of varying individual perspectives on physical activity, Bleich asked him how that diversity can be reconciled with the application of systems science approaches. Jakicic reiterated that viewing physical activity as exercise is a barrier for some people, and that certain forms of physical activity requiring greater financial investment or higher fitness levels are less accessible. He called for a broad scope of activity options to reach the greatest number of people.

### Engaging the Private Sector

Bleich next asked the speakers about ideas for engaging the private sector in obesity prevention. Allender suggested inviting business owners and leaders to contribute as members of the community, as well as including businesses in trial design. As an example of the latter, he referenced initiatives in which supermarket efforts to modify food presentation and marketing have resulted in changes in purchasing patterns. He shared his experience with a ready and willing business community, urging others not to overlook this powerful resource. Spring mentioned the existence of obesity interventions in large worksites and highlighted the American Heart Association's CEO Roundtable, a leadership collaborative dedicated to implementing evidence-based approaches to workplace health that focus on engaging employees and building a corporate culture of health. She also pointed to a tremendous interest in commercializing health interventions, which she identified as an opportunity for beneficial dialogue with potential collaborators.

### Lessons from Community Engagement

The final question solicited the three speakers' thoughts on how engagement with communities has influenced their research priorities and study designs. Jakicic described a needs analysis that was conducted in a community before an intervention was developed, explaining that it helped researchers identify respected individuals perceived by community members as core leaders. The experience helped the researchers understand how best to engage the community, he recalled, and identified key influencers with whom researchers should partner. Spring stressed the importance of cultivating humility and trust so it is clear that researchers understand the community's needs. Allender called for researchers to recognize that their role is to provide tools and opportunities for communities to solve problems in the way that makes sense for them.

## CLOSING REMARKS FOR PART II

Christina Economos, co-founder and director of ChildObesity180 and professor and New Balance chair in childhood nutrition in the Friedman School of Nutrition Science at Tufts University, reflected on themes that had emerged from the workshop presentations and discussions. She highlighted examples of structural and social drivers with the potential to shape public health and offer opportunities for systems change as they relate to obesity solutions, including context, inequities, structural racism, disparities, bias, power dynamics, relationships, mindset, trust, humility, engagement, multilevel interventions, and technology. Nicolaas Pronk, president of HealthPartners Institute, chief science officer at HealthPartners, and chair of the Roundtable on Obesity Solutions, shared his takeaways from the workshop, emphasizing the importance of leadership, humility, community engagement, stakeholder involvement, building trust, and appreciating complexity as crucial to progress and impact. Pronk ended Part II of the workshop with a preview of the roundtable's September 2020 workshop. He indicated that although both qualitative (e.g., mapping) and quantitative (e.g., modeling) systems science approaches are important, the follow-on workshop will focus on modeling of various approaches that could guide future obesity research and action and on support structures for those approaches.

# References

Aral, S., and C. Nicolaides. 2017. Exercise contagion in a global social network. *Nature Communications* 8:14753. https://doi.org/10.1038/ncomms14753.

Auchincloss, A. H., and A. V. Diez Roux. 2008. A new tool for epidemiology: The usefulness of dynamic-agent models in understanding place effects on health. *American Journal of Epidemiology* 168:1–8.

Auchincloss, A. H., R. L. Riolo., D. G. Brown, J. Cook, and A. V. Diez Roux. 2011. An agent-based model of income inequalities in diet in the context of residential segregation. *American Journal of Preventive Medicine* 40(3):303–311. https://doi.org/10.1016/j.amepre.2010.10.033.

Auerbach, D. M., W. W. Darrow, H. W. Jaffe, and J. W. Curran. 1984. Cluster of cases of the acquired immune deficiency syndrome: Patients linked by sexual contact. *American Journal of Medicine* 76(3):487–492. doi: 10.1016/0002-9343(84)90668-5.

Benjamin, R. 2019. *Race after technology: Abolitionist tools for the new Jim Code (1st Ed.)*. Medford, MA: Polity Press.

Calancie, L., K. Fullerton, J. M. Appel, A. R. Korn, E. Hennessy, P. Hovmand, and C. D. Economos. 2020. Implementing group model building with the Shape Up Under 5 Community committee working to prevent early childhood obesity in Somerville, Massachusetts. *Journal of Public Health Management and Practice*. doi: 10.1097/PHH.0000000000001213.

Ceasar, J. N., C. Ayers, M. R. Andrews, S. E. Claudel, K. Tamura, S. Das, J. de Lemos, I. J. Neeland, T. M. Powell-Wiley. 2020. Unfavorable perceived neighborhood environment associates with less routine healthcare utilization: Data from the Dallas Heart Study. *PLOS ONE* 15(3):e0230041.

Centola, D. 2011. An experimental study of homophily in the adoption of health behavior. *Science* 334:1269–1272.

Christakis, N. A., and J. H. Fowler. 2007. The spread of obesity in a large social network over 32 years. *New England Journal of Medicine* 357(4):370–379. doi: 10.1056/NEJMsa066082.

Davis, M. M., S. Nambiar, M. E. Mayorga, E. Sullivan, K. Hicklin, M. C. O'Leary, K. Dillon, K. H. Lich, Y. Gu, and B. K. Lind. 2019. Mailed FIT (fecal immunochemical test), navigation or patient reminders? Using microsimulation to inform selection of interventions to increase colorectal cancer screening in Medicaid enrollees. *Preventive Medicine* 129:105836.

de la Haye, K., G. Robins, P. Mohr, and C. Wilson. 2011. Homophily and contagion as explanations for weight similarities among adolescent friends. *Journal of Adolescent Health* 49(4):421–427. doi: 10.1016/j.jadohealth.2011.02.008.

de la Haye, K., B. M. Bell, and S. J. Salvy. 2019. The role of maternal social networks on the outcomes of a home-based childhood obesity prevention pilot intervention. *Journal of Social Structures* 20(3):7–28. doi: 10.21307/joss-2019-004.

Ennett, S. T., and K. E. Bauman. 1993. Peer group structure and adolescent cigarette smoking: A social network analysis. *Journal of Health and Social Behavior* 34(3):226–236.

Epstein, J. 2008. Why model? *Journal of Artificial Societies and Social Simulation* 11(4):12. http://jasss.soc.surrey.ac.uk/11/4/12.html.

Flórez, K. R., B. Bell, and K. de la Haye. 2020. *Unraveling the relationship between food insecurity, acculturation, and diet quality in Mexican Americans: What is the role of social networks.* http://www.pfeffer.at/sunbelt/talks/1142.html (accessed January 29, 2021).

Ford, C. L., and C. O. Airhihenbuwa. 2010a. Critical race theory, race equity, and public health: Toward antiracism praxis. *American Journal of Public Health* 100(Suppl 1):S30–S35. doi: 10.2105/AJPH.2009.171058.

Ford, C. L., and C. O. Airhihenbuwa. 2010b. The public health critical race methodology: Praxis for antiracism research. *Social Science and Medicine* 71(8):1390–1398. doi: 10.1016/j.socscimed.2010.07.030.

Ford, C. L., and C. O. Airhihenbuwa. 2018. Commentary: Just what is critical race theory and what's it doing in a progressive field like public health? *Ethnicity and Disease* 28(Suppl 1):223–230. doi:10.18865/ed.28.S1.223.

Ford, C. L., L. M. Takahashi, P. P. Chandanabhumma, M. E. Ruiz, and W. E. Cunningham. 2018. Anti-racism methods for big data research: Lessons learned from the HIV testing, linkage, & retention in care (HIV TLR) study. *Ethnicity and Disease* 28(Suppl 1):261–266.

Frerichs, L., K. H. Lich, G. Dave, and G. Corbie-Smith. 2016. Integrating systems science and community-based participatory research to achieve health equity. *American Journal of Public Health* 106(2):215–222.

Gillman, M. W., and R. A. Hammond. 2016. Precision treatment and precision prevention: Integrating below and above the skin. *JAMA Pediatrics* 170(1):9–10.

Hammond, R. A. 2009. Complex systems modeling for obesity research. *Preventing Chronic Disease* 6(3):A97. http://www.cdc.gov/pcd/issues/2009/jul/09_0017.htm.

Hammond, R. A., J. T. Ornstein, L. K. Fellows, L. Dubé, R. Levitan, and A. Dagher. 2012. A model of food reward learning with dynamic reward exposure. *Frontiers in Computational Neuroscience* 6:82. https://doi.org/10.3389/fncom.2012.00082.

Hennessy, E., C. Economos, and R. A. Hammond (with the SUS Map Team and the COMPACT Team). 2020. Integrating complex systems methods to advance obesity prevention intervention research. *Health Education & Behavior* 47(2):213–223.

IOM (Institute of Medicine). 2012. *Accelerating progress in obesity prevention: Solving the weight of the nation.* Washington, DC: The National Academies Press. https://doi.org/10.17226/13275.

IOM. 2015. *Assessing the use of agent-based models for tobacco regulation.* Washington, DC: The National Academies Press. https://doi.org/10.17226/19018.

IOM and NRC (National Research Council). 2015. *A framework for assessing effects of the food system.* Washington, DC: The National Academies Press. https://doi.org/10.17226/18846.

Jones, C. P. 2000. Levels of racism: A theoretic framework and a gardener's tale. *American Journal of Public Health* 90(8):1212–1215. doi:10.2105/ajph.90.8.1212.

Kania, J., M. Kramer, and P. Senge. 2018. *The water of systems change.* Boston, MA: FSG.

Kasman, M., R. A. Hammond, B. Heuberger, A. Mack-Crane, R. Purcell, C. Economos, B. Swinburn, S. Allender, and M. Nichols. 2019. Activating a community: An agent-based model of romp and chomp, a whole-of-community childhood obesity intervention. *Obesity* 27(9):1494–1502.

Keyes, K. M., and S. Galea. 2016. *Population health science.* Oxford, UK: Oxford University Press.

Kindig, D., and G. Stoddart. 2003. What is population health? *American Journal of Public Health* 93:380–383. https://dx.doi.org/10.2105%2Fajph.93.3.380.

Koehly, L. M., and A. Loscalzo. 2009. Adolescent obesity and social networks. *Preventing Chronic Disease* 6(3):A99.

Korn, A. R., E. Hennessy, A. Tovar, C. Finn, R. A. Hammond, and C. D. Economos. 2018. Engaging coalitions in community-based childhood obesity prevention interventions: A mixed methods assessment. *Childhood Obesity* 14(8):537–552.

Kumanyika, S. K. 2019. A framework for increasing equity impact in obesity prevention. *American Journal of Public Health* 109(10):1350–1357. https://doi.org/10.2105/AJPH.2019.305221.

Langellier, B., K. Lobban, U. Bilal, F. Montes, J. Meisel, L. O. Cardoso, and R. A. Hammond. 2019. Complex systems approaches to diet: A systematic review. *American Journal of Preventive Medicine* 57(2):273–281.

Luke, D. A., and K. A. Stamatakis. 2012. Systems science methods in public health: Dynamics, networks, and agents. *Annual Review of Public Health* 33:357–376. doi: 10.1146/annurev-publhealth-031210-101222.

Mabry, P. L., and R. M. Bures. 2014. Systems science for obesity-related research questions: An introduction to the theme issue. *American Journal of Public Health* 104(7):1157–1159. doi: 10.2105/AJPH.2014.302083.

Mabry, P. L., S. E. Marcus, P. I. Clark, S. J. Leischow, and D. Mendez. 2010. Systems science: A revolution in public health policy research. *American Journal of Public Health* 100(7):1161–1163. doi: 10.2105/AJPH.2010.198176.

Marshall, B. D. L., and S. Galea. 2015. Formalizing the role of complex systems methods in causal inference and epidemiology. *American Journal of Epidemiology* 181(2):92–99. https://doi.org/10.1093/aje/kwu274.

McGlashan, J., K. de la Haye, P. Wang, and S. Allender. 2019. Collaboration in complex systems: Multilevel network analysis for community-based obesity prevention interventions. *Scientific Reports* 9:1.

Meadows, D. 1999. *Leverage points: Places to intervene in a system.* Hartland, VT: The Sustainability Institute.

Morshed, A. B., M. Kasman, B. Heuberger, R. A. Hammond, and P. S. Hovmand. 2019. A systematic review of system dynamics and agent-based obesity models: Evaluating obesity as part of the global syndemic. *Obesity Reviews* 2019:1–18.

Mustafa, A. S. 2020. *Ward 8 community economic development planning process.* https://www.ward8cedplan.com/our-plan (accessed January 29, 2021).

NASEM (National Academies of Sciences, Engineering, and Medicine). 2016. *Assessing prevalence and trends in obesity: Navigating the evidence.* Washington, DC: The National Academies Press. https://doi.org/10.17226/23505.

Nianogo, R. A., and A. A. Onyebuchi. 2015. Agent-based modeling of noncommunicable diseases: A systematic review. *American Journal of Public Health* 105(3):e20–e31.

Noble, S. U. 2018. *Algorithms of oppression: How search engines reinforce racism (1st Ed.).* New York: New York University Press.

Ogden, C. L., M. D. Carroll, M. A. McDowell, and K. M. Flegal. 2007. Obesity among adults in the United States—No statistically significant change since 2003–2004. *NCHS data brief no. 1.* Hyattsville, MD: National Center for Health Statistics.

Powell, W., L. Frerichs, R. Townsley, M. Mayorga, J. Richmond, G. Corbie-Smith, S. Wheeler, and K. Hassmiller Lich. 2020. The potential impact of the Affordable Care Act and Medicaid expansion on reducing colorectal cancer screening disparities in African American males. *PLOS ONE* 15(1):e0226942.

Powell-Wiley, T. M., K. Moore, N. Allen, R. Block, K. R. Evenson, M. Mujahid, and A. V. Diez Roux. 2017a. Associations of neighborhood crime and safety and with changes in body mass index and waist circumference: The Multi-Ethnic Study of Atherosclerosis. *American Journal of Epidemiology* 186(3):280–288. doi:10.1093/aje/kwx082.

Powell-Wiley, T. M., M. S. Wong, J. Adu-Brimpong, S. T. Brown, D. L. Hertenstein, E. Zenkov, M. C. Ferguson, S. Thomas, D. Sampson, C. Ahuja, J. Rivers, and B. Y. Lee. 2017b. Simulating the impact of crime on African American women's physical activity and obesity. *Obesity* 25(12). https://doi.org/10.1002/oby.22040.

Quistberg, D. A., A. V. Diez Roux, U. Bilal. K. Moore, A. Ortigoza, D. A. Rodriguez, O. L. Sarmiento, P. Frenz, A. A. Friche, W. T. Caiaffa, A. Vives, J. J. Miranda, and the SALURBAL Group. 2018. Building a data platform for cross-country urban health studies: the SALURBAL Study. *Journal of Urban Health* 96:311–337. https://doi.org/10.1007/s11524-018-00326-0.

Reardon, S. F., R. Baker, M. Kasman, D. Klasik, and J. B. Townsend. 2018. What levels of racial diversity can be achieved with socioeconomic-based affirmative action? Evidence from a simulation model. *Journal of Policy Analysis and Management* 37(3):630–657.

Rose, G. 1985. Sick individuals and sick populations. *International Journal of Epidemiology* 14(1):32–38. https://doi.org/10.1093/ije/14.1.32.

Roser, M. 2017. Link between health spending and life expectancy: The US is an outlier. https://ourworldindata.org/the-link-between-life-expectancy-and-health-spending-us-focus (accessed January 28, 2021).

Schaefer, D. R. and S. D. Simpkins. 2014. Using social network analysis to clarify the role of obesity in selection of adolescent friends. *American Journal of Public Health* 104(7):1223–1229. https://doi.org/10.2105/AJPH.2013.301768.

Schaefer, D., S. D. Simpkins, A. E. Vest, C. Price, and S. Simpkins-Chaput. 2011. The role of extracurricular activities in developing and maintaining adolescent friendships: New insights through social network analysis. *Developmental Psychology* 4:1141–1152.

Schraefel, M. C., and E. Hekler. 2020. Tuning: An approach for supporting healthful adaptation. *Interactions* 27(2):48–53.

Secretary's Advisory Committee for Healthy People 2030. 2018. Issue briefs to inform development and implementation of Healthy People 2030. https://www.healthypeople.gov/sites/default/files/HP2030_Committee-Combined-Issue%20Briefs_2019-508c.pdf (accessed January 28, 2021).

Simpkins, S. D., A. E. Vest, and C. D. Price. 2011. Intergenerational continuity and discontinuity in Mexican-origin youths' participation in organized activities: Insights from mixed-methods. *Journal of Family Psychology* 25(6):814–824. doi: 10.1037/a0025853.

Spring, B., A. F. Pfammatter, S. H. Marchese, T. Stump, C. Pellegrini, H. G. McFadden, D. Hedeker, J. Siddique, N. Jordan, and L. M. Collins. 2020. A factorial experiment to optimize remotely delivered behavioral treatment for obesity: Results of the Opt-IN Study. *Obesity* 28(9).

Swinburn, B. A., V. I. Kraak, S. Allender, V. J. Atkins, P. I. Baker, J. R. Bogard, H. Brinsden, A. Calvillo, O. De Schutter, R. Devarajan, M. Ezzati, S. Friel, S. Goenka, R. A. Hammond, G. Hastings, C. Hawkes, M. Herrero, P. S. Hovmand, M. Howden, L. M. Jaacks, A. B. Kapetanaki, M. Kasman, H. V. Kuhnlein, S. K. Kumanyika, B. Larijani, T. Lobstein, M. W. Long, V. K. R. Matsudo, S. D. H. Mills, G. Morgan, A. Morshed, P. M. Nece, A. Pan, D. W. Patterson, G. Sacks, M. Shekar, G. L. Simmons, W. Smit, A. Tootee, S. Vandevijvere, W. E. Waterlander, L. Wolfenden, and W. H. Dietz. 2019. The Global Syndemic of Obesity, Undernutrition, and Climate Change: The Lancet Commission report. *The Lancet* 393(10173):791–846.

Trogdon, J. G., J. Nonnemaker, and J. Pais. 2008. Peer effects in adolescent overweight. *Journal of Health Economics* 27(5):1388–1399. https://doi.org/10.1016/j.jhealeco.2008.05.003.

United Kingdom Government Office for Science. 2007. *Tackling obesities: Future choices—Obesity system atlas.* London: Government Office for Science. https://assets.publishing.service.gov.uk/government/uploads/system/uploads/attachment_data/file/295153/07-1177-obesity-system-atlas.pdf (accessed January 28, 2021).

Weiner, B. J., M. A. Lewis, S. B. Clauser, and K. B. Stitzenberg. 2012. In search of synergy: Strategies for combining interventions at multiple levels. *Journal of the National Cancer Institute Monographs* 2012(44):34–41.

Wood, W., and D. T. Neal. 2016. Healthy through habit: Interventions for initiating & maintaining health behavior change. *Behavioral Science & Policy* 2(1):71–83.

Valente, T. W. 2012. Network interventions. *Science* 337(6090):49–53. doi: 10.1126/science.1217330.

Valente, T. W., K. Fujimoto, C. P. Chou, and D. Spruijt-Metz. 2009. Adolescent affiliations and adiposity: A social network analysis of friendships and obesity. *Journal of Adolescent Health* 45(2):202–204. doi: 10.1016/j.jadohealth.2009.01.007.

Zhang, S., K. de la Haye, M. Ji, and R. An. 2018. Applications of social network analysis to obesity: A systematic review. *Obesity Etiology.* https://doi.org/10.1111/obr.12684.

# Appendix A

# Workshop Agendas

**PART I**

**Integrating Systems and Sectors Toward Obesity Solutions:
A Virtual Workshop**

Monday, April 6, 2020
9:00 AM–12 PM ET
Zoom: https://nasem.zoom.us/j/730323933

**Introduction and Overview of Systems Theories,
Methodologies, and Applications**
Objective: Provide background on systems theories, methodologies, and applications.

9:00 AM    **Welcome**
           *Nico Pronk, Chair, Roundtable on Obesity Solutions*

9:10       **Overview/History of Systems Science**
           *Ross Hammond, Washington University in St. Louis*

9:40       **Thinking in Systems to Address Health Inequities and Improve
           Population Health**
           *Sandro Galea, Boston University*

10:10    **Overview of Applications**
*Douglas Luke, Washington University in St. Louis*

10:40    **Break**

10:50    **Panel Discussion**
*Moderator: Daniel E. Rivera, Arizona State University*

11:25    **Audience Q&A**
*Moderator: Daniel E. Rivera, Arizona State University*

11:50    **Closing Remarks**
*Chris Economos, Co-Vice Chair, Roundtable on Obesity
Solutions*

12:00 PM    **Virtual Workshop Adjourns**

## PART II

Tuesday, June 30, 2020
10:00 AM–3:15 PM ET

10:00 AM    **Welcome and Summary of April 6 Virtual Workshop**
*Nico Pronk, Chair, and Chris Economos, Co-Vice Chair,
Roundtable on Obesity Solutions*

**Session 1—Complex Systems in Society and the Context for Obesity**
Objective: Explore systems and contributing factors that can influence
obesity.

10:15    **Power Dynamics, Structural Racism, and Relationships**
*Moderator: Shiriki Kumanyika, Drexel University*

*Chandra Ford, University of California, Los Angeles
Kayla de la Haye, University of Southern California*

**Panel Discussion and Audience Q&A**

11:00       **Resources, Place-Based Issues, Policy, and Political Will**
*Moderator: Giselle Corbie-Smith, University of North Carolina at Chapel Hill*

*Ana Diez Roux, Drexel University*
*Tiffany Powell-Wiley, National Heart, Lung, and Blood Institute, National Institutes of Health*

**Panel Discussion and Audience Q&A**

**Session 2—Impacting Complex Systems That Can Influence Obesity**
Objective: Explore how systems may influence obesity. Consider opportunities for systems change as they relate to obesity solutions.

12:00 PM    **Participatory Nature of Interventions and Education**
*Moderator: Sara Czaja, Weill Cornell Medicine*

*Leah Frerichs, University of North Carolina at Chapel Hill*
*Matt Kasman, Brookings Institution*

**Panel Discussion and Audience Q&A**

12:45       **Obesity-Related Opportunities for Systems Change**
*Moderator: Ihuoma Eneli, Nationwide Children's Hospital*

*Eric Hekler, University of California, San Diego*
*Erin Hennessy, Tufts University*

**Panel Discussion and Audience Q&A**

1:30        **Lunch**

**SESSION 3—Examples from the Field: Applying Systems Thinking to Population Health Issues**

Objective: Demonstrate how research studies are exploring the application of systems thinking to address obesity and the health and well-being of the population.

2:00        *Moderator: Sara Bleich, Harvard T.H. Chan School of Public Health*

            *John Jakicic, University of Pittsburgh*
            *Bonnie Spring, Northwestern University*
            *Steve Allender, Deakin University*

            **Audience Q&A**

3:00        **Wrap-Up Comments**
            *Nico Pronk and Chris Economos*

3:15        **Adjourn**

# Appendix B

# Acronyms and Abbreviations

AJPH        *American Journal of Public Health*

BMI         body mass index

CHD         coronary heart disease
COMPACT     Childhood Obesity Modeling for Prevention and Community
            Transformation
CRT         critical race theory

DPP         Diabetes Prevention Program

HIV TLR     Human Immunodeficiency Virus Testing, Linkage and
            Retention in care

MIDAS       Models of Infectious Disease Agent Study

NHANES      National Health and Nutrition Examination Survey
NIH         National Institutes of Health

RCT         randomized controlled trial

SALURBAL    Salud Urbana en America Latina

# Appendix C

# Glossary

**Agent-based modeling** uses computer simulation to study complex systems from the ground up by examining how individual elements of a system (agents) behave as a function of individual properties, their environment, and their interactions with each other. Through these behaviors, emergent properties of the overall system are revealed (Luke and Stamatakis, 2012).

**Community-based system dynamics** differs from other group model building or participatory modeling approaches because of its explicit focus on developing systems thinking capabilities among community members, including an endogenous or feedback perspective, an appreciation for nonlinear system behavior, and an emphasis on operational thinking (Hovmand, 2014).

**Complex systems** are made up of heterogeneous elements that interact with each other. The interactions of these elements produce a unique effect that is different from the effects of the individual elements alone (Gallagher and Appenzeller, 1999).

**Group model building** is a participatory approach that is used to build the capacity of a group to use systems thinking to develop causal loop diagrams and other system dynamics models (Siokou et al., 2014).

**Network analysis** is a research method and scientific paradigm that focuses on the relationships among sets of actors. The actors can be any type of entity that can have a relationship or tie with other entities (e.g., persons, animals, organizations, countries, websites, documents, and even genes) (Luke and Stamatakis, 2012).

**Stepped wedge cluster randomized trials** involve the collection of observations during a baseline period in which no clusters are exposed to the intervention. Following this, at regular intervals, or steps, a cluster (or group of clusters) is randomized to receive the intervention (Brown and Lilford, 2006; Mdege et al., 2011), and all participants are once again measured (Hussey and Hughes, 2007). This process continues until all clusters have received the intervention. Finally, one more measurement is made after all clusters have received the intervention.

**System dynamics** is based on the premise that complex behaviors of a system result from the interplay of feedback loops, stocks and flows, and delays. The focus is on building models to represent the dynamic complexity of collective, often high-level phenomena (Luke and Stamatakis, 2012).

**Systems science approaches** are a broad class of analytical approaches that aim to uncover the behavior of complex systems. A distinction is made between hard systems methods (e.g., quantitative dynamic model building) and soft systems methods (e.g., qualitative, action-based research methods) (Carey et al., 2015).

**Systems thinking** is a broad paradigm concerned with interrelationships, perspectives, and boundaries (Williams and Hummelbrunner, 2011).

## REFERENCES

Brown, C. A., and R. J. Lilford. 2006. The stepped wedge trial design: A systematic review. *BMC Medical Research Methodology* 6:54.

Carey, G., E. Malbon, N. Carey, A. Joyce, B. Crammond, and A. Carey. 2015. Systems science and systems thinking for public health: A systematic review of the field. *British Medical Journal Open* 5(12):e009002.

Gallagher, R., and T. Appenzeller. 1999. Beyond reductionism. *Science* 284:79.

Hovmand, P. 2014. *Community based system dynamics.* New York: Springer-Verlag.

Hussey, M. A., and J. P. Hughes. 2007. Design and analysis of stepped wedge cluster randomized trials. *Contemporary Clinical Trials* 28(2):182–191.

Luke, D. A., and K. A. Stamatakis. 2012. Systems science methods in public health: Dynamics, networks, and agents. *Annual Review of Public Health* 33:357–376.

Mdege, N. D., M.-S. Man, C. A. Taylor, and D. J. Torgerson. 2011. Systematic review of stepped wedge cluster randomized trials shows that design is particularly used to evaluate interventions during routine implementation. *Journal of Clinical Epidemiology* 64(9):936–948.

Siokou, C., R. Morgan, and A. Shiell. 2014. Group model building: A participatory approach to understanding and acting on systems. *Public Health Research & Practice* 25(1):e2511404.

Williams, B., and R. Hummelbrunner. 2011. *Systems concepts in action: A practitioner's toolkit.* Stanford, CA: Stanford University Press.

# Appendix D

# Biographical Sketches of Workshop Speakers and Planning Committee Members

**Steven Allender, Ph.D.,** is a professor of public health and the founding director of the Global Obesity Centre (GLOBE) at Deakin University. GLOBE is a World Health Organization (WHO) Collaborating Centre for Obesity Prevention that supports efforts to improve health in more than 30 countries worldwide and works directly with WHO to achieve these aims. Dr. Allender has an ongoing program of research on solving complex problems concerning the burden of chronic disease and obesity prevention. His recent work has focused on the burden of chronic disease, malnutrition, and climate change in developed and developing countries and the possibilities for using complex systems approaches for community-based intervention. Dr. Allender leads two partnership grants from Australia's National Health and Medical Research Council on community-based childhood obesity strategies, he is a lead investigator for the Centre of Research Excellence in Food Retail Environments for Health and the European Union Horizon 2020 CO-CREATE grant for healthier policy in Europe, and he is a named researcher for the Australian Prevention Partnership Centre. He has received lead investigator funding from several organizations, including the U.S. National Institutes of Health, the National Health and Medical Research Council of Australia, the Australian Heart Foundation, VicHealth, the British Heart Foundation, the Western Alliance, the European Heart Foundation, and the European Union. Dr. Allender holds a Ph.D. from the University of Ballarat.

**Sara N. Bleich, Ph.D.,** is a professor of public health policy at the Harvard T.H. Chan School of Public Health in the university's Department of Health

Policy and Management. She is also the Carol K. Pforzheimer professor at the Radcliffe Institute for Advanced Study and a member of the faculty at the Harvard Kennedy School of Government. Her research provides evidence to support policy alternatives for obesity prevention and control, particularly among populations at higher risk for obesity. A signature theme throughout her work is an interest in asking simple, meaningful questions about the complex problem of obesity, which can fill important gaps in the literature. Dr. Bleich has received multiple awards, including one for excellence in public interest communication from the Frank Conference at the University of Florida. She was also a White House fellow, serving as a senior policy advisor to the U.S. Department of Agriculture and the Let's Move initiative of First Lady Michelle Obama. Dr. Bleich holds a B.A. in psychology from Columbia University and a Ph.D. in health policy from Harvard University.

**Giselle Corbie-Smith, M.Sc., M.D.,** is the Kenan distinguished professor in the Departments of Social Medicine and Medicine and the director of the Center for Health Equity Research at the University of North Carolina (UNC) School of Medicine. She has served as the principal investigator of several community-based participatory research projects focused on disease risk reduction among rural racial and ethnic minorities. These projects have been supported by the National Heart, Lung, and Blood Institute; the Robert Wood Johnson Foundation (RWJF); the National Center for Minority Health and Health Disparities; the National Institute of Nursing Research; The Greenwall Foundation; and the National Human Genome Research Institute. Dr. Corbie-Smith is committed to drawing communities, faculty, and health care providers into working partnerships in clinical and translational research: this engagement ultimately transforms the way that academic investigators and community members interact while boosting public trust in research. She is also deeply committed to working in North Carolina by bringing research to communities, involving community members as partners in research, and improving the health of minority populations and underserved areas. In 2013 she established and became the director of the UNC Center for Health Equity Research to bring together collaborative multidisciplinary teams of scholars, trainees, and community members to improve North Carolina communities' health through a shared commitment to innovation, collaboration, and health equity. Dr. Corbie-Smith is currently the co–principal investigator for the Advancing Change Leadership Clinical Scholars Program of RWJF, which provides intensive learning, collaboration, networking, and leadership development to seasoned clinicians to create a community of practitioners promoting health equity across the country. She recently served as the president of the Society of General Internal Medicine. She is an elected member of the

National Academy of Medicine. Dr. Corbie-Smith holds an M.Sc. in clinical research from Emory University and an M.D. from the Albert Einstein College of Medicine.

**Sara J. Czaja, M.S., Ph.D.,** is a professor of gerontology and the director of the Center on Aging and Behavioral Research in the Division of Geriatrics and Palliative Medicine at Weill Cornell Medicine. She is also an emeritus professor of psychiatry and behavioral sciences at the University of Miami Miller School of Medicine, where she previously served as the director of the Center on Aging. Dr. Czaja is also the director of the multisite Center for Research and Education on Aging and Technology Enhancement of the National Institutes of Health and the co-director of the Center for Enhancing Neurocognitive Health, Abilities, Networks, & Community Engagement of the National Institute on Disability, Independent Living, and Rehabilitation Research. Her research interests include aging and cognition, caregiving, aging and technology, aging and work, training, and functional assessment. She has received long-term research support from the National Institutes of Health and other agencies and has published extensively on these topics. She is a fellow of the American Psychological Association (APA), the Human Factors and Ergonomics Society, and the Gerontological Society of American. She is a past president of APA's Division 20 (adult development and aging) and has served as a member of the Board on Human Systems Integration of the National Academies of Sciences, Engineering, and Medicine; as a member of the Institute of Medicine (IOM) Committee on the Public Health Dimensions of Cognitive Aging; and as a member of the IOM Committee on Family Caring for Older Adults. Dr. Czaja is a recipient of the M. Powell Lawton Distinguished Contribution Award for Applied Gerontology from APA; the Social Impact Award of the Association of Computing Machinery, and the Franklin V. Taylor Award from APA's Division 21 (applied experimental and engineering psychology). She is also a recipient of the Jack A. Kraft Award for Innovation from the Human Factors and Ergonomics Society, APA's prize for interdisciplinary team research, and the Richard Kalish Innovative Book Publication Award of the Gerontological Society of America. Dr. Czaja holds an M.S. and a Ph.D. in industrial engineering from the State University of New York University at Buffalo.

**Kayla de la Haye, Ph.D.,** is an assistant professor of preventive medicine at the University of Southern California. She works to promote health and prevent disease by applying social network analysis and systems science. Her research, funded by the National Institutes of Health, the National Science Foundation, and the Department of Defense, targets family and community social networks to promote healthy eating and prevent childhood obesity.

She also studies the role of social networks and systems in group problem solving in families, teams, and coalitions. Dr. de la Haye is the treasurer of the International Network of Social Network Analysis (INSNA) and a recipient of the INSNA Freeman award for significant contributions to the study of social structure. She holds a Ph.D. in psychology from the University of Adelaide, Australia.

**Ana Diez Roux, M.D., M.P.H., Ph.D.,** is the dean and the distinguished university professor of epidemiology in the Dornsife School of Public Health at Drexel University. Before joining Drexel, she served on the faculties of Columbia University and the University of Michigan, where she was the chair of the Department of Epidemiology and the director of the Center for Social Epidemiology and Population Health at the university's School of Public Health. Dr. Diez Roux focuses on the social determinants of population health and the study of how neighborhoods affect health, and has been highly influential in the policy debates on population health and its determinants. Her research areas include social epidemiology and health disparities, environmental health effects, urban health, psychosocial factors in health, cardiovascular disease epidemiology, and the use of multilevel methods. Recent areas of work include social environment–gene interactions and the use of complex systems approaches in population health. Dr. Diez Roux has led large research and training programs in the United States and in collaboration with various institutions in Latin America with support from the National Institutes of Health (NIH) and several foundations. She has been a member of the MacArthur Foundation's Network on Socioeconomic Factors and Health and was the co-director of the NIH-sponsored Network on Inequality, Complexity, and Health. Dr. Diez Roux holds an M.D. from the University of Buenos Aires and an M.P.H. and a Ph.D. from the Johns Hopkins School of Hygiene and Public Health.

**Christina (Chris) Economos, M.S., Ph.D.,** holds the New Balance chair in childhood nutrition and is the chair of the Division of Nutrition Interventions, Communication, & Behavior Change at the Friedman School of Nutrition Science and Policy and Medical School at Tufts University. She leads a research team using a systems approach to study behavioral interventions, strategic communications, and promotion of physical activity to reduce childhood obesity. She has authored more than 150 scientific publications and is also the co-founder and the director of ChildObesity180, a unique organization that brings together leaders from diverse disciplines to generate urgency and find solutions to the childhood obesity epidemic. Dr. Economos is involved in national obesity and public health activities and has served on four committees of the National Academies of Sciences, Engineering, and Medicine, including the Roundtable on Obesity Solutions and the Committee on an Evidence-Based Framework for Obesity Prevention Decision Making. She holds a B.S. from Boston University, an M.S. in applied physiology and nutrition from Columbia University, and a Ph.D. in nutritional biochemistry from Tufts University.

**Ihuoma Eneli, M.S., M.D.,** is a board-certified general pediatrician, a professor of clinical pediatrics at The Ohio State University College of Medicine, and the director of the Nationwide Children's Hospital Center for Healthy Weight and Nutrition (CHWN). She is also an associate director for the American Academy of Pediatrics Institute for the Healthy Childhood Weight. In her role as the CHWN director, Dr. Eneli oversees a comprehensive tertiary care pediatric obesity center with activities that include advocacy, prevention, medical weight management, and adolescent bariatric surgery. She also directs the Primary Care Obesity Network, which provides obesity-related training, resources, and community integration for primary care practices in central Ohio. Her research, funded by the National Institutes of Health (NIH) and other sources, focuses particularly on intervention research for pediatric obesity, and she has authored several publications and book chapters in her field. Dr. Eneli holds an M.D. from the University of Nigeria and an M.S. in epidemiology from Michigan State University, where she completed her pediatric residency, served as chief resident, and completed an NIH-K30 institutional clinical research fellowship.

**Chandra Ford, M.P.H., Ph.D.,** is an associate professor of community health sciences and the founding director of the Center for the Study of Racism, Social Justice & Health at the University of California, Los Angeles (UCLA). Prior to joining UCLA, she completed postdoctoral training in social medicine at the University of North Carolina at Chapel Hill and in epidemiology at the Columbia University Mailman School of Public Health, where she was a W.K. Kellogg Foundation Kellogg Health Scholar. Dr. Ford's research examines relationships between racism-related factors and disparities in the HIV care continuum and advances the conceptual and methodological tools for studying racism's relationship to health disparities. She is a member of the Minority Affairs Committee of the American College of Epidemiology and the chair of the Faculty Advisory Committee of the Ralph J. Bunche Center for African American Studies at UCLA. She previously served as a member of the Committee on Community-Based Solutions to Promote Health Equity in the United States of the National Academies of Sciences, Engineering, and Medicine and as the co-chair of the Committee on Science of the Anti-Racism Collaborative of the American Public Health Association. She also previously served as the president of the Society for the Analysis of African American Public Health Issues. Dr.

Ford holds an M.P.H. from the University of Pittsburgh and a Ph.D. from the University of North Carolina.

**Leah Frerichs, M.S., Ph.D.,** is an assistant professor in the Department of Health Policy and Management at the University of North Carolina at Chapel Hill. As a public health researcher and practitioner with expertise in community-based participatory and systems science research, her research involves community-based program planning, evaluation, and research with diverse communities, including American Indian, Latino, and African American populations. She integrates engaged and participatory research approaches with systems science methods in order to address health issues in underserved communities. She uses visual diagramming and facilitated interactions with computer models to improve understanding of the complex dynamics influencing health problems of interest and to improve the implementation and dissemination of optimal combinations of interventions and policies. Dr. Frerichs holds an M.S. in community and behavioral health from The University of Iowa and a Ph.D. in health promotion and disease prevention research from the University of Nebraska Medical Center.

**Sandro Galea, M.D.,** is the dean and the Robert A. Knox professor at the Boston University School of Public Health. He previously held academic and leadership positions at Columbia University, the University of Michigan, and The New York Academy of Medicine. He has published extensively and is a regular contributor to a range of public media on the social causes of health, mental health, and the consequences of trauma. Dr. Galea has been listed as one of the most widely cited scholars in the social sciences. He is the chair of the board of the Association of Schools and Programs of Public Health and the past president of the Society for Epidemiologic Research and of the Interdisciplinary Association for Population Health Science. He is an elected member of the National Academy of Medicine and he has received several lifetime achievement awards. Dr. Galea holds an M.D. from the University of Toronto, graduate degrees from Harvard University and Columbia University, and an honorary doctorate from the University of Glasgow.

**Ross Hammond, Ph.D.,** is the Betty Bofinger Brown associate professor at Washington University in St. Louis. His research applies complex systems tools to generate new insights into the social dynamics that drive many difficult policy problems, as well as to identify potential leverage points or windows for intervention. He is a senior fellow in economic studies at the Brookings Institution, where he is the director of the Center on Social Dynamics and Policy. He also holds academic appointments at the

Harvard T.H. Chan School of Public Health and the Santa Fe Institute. Dr. Hammond is an appointed member of the advisory council of the National Institute on Minority Health and Health Disparities advisory council; a public health advisor for the National Cancer Institute; an advisory special government employee for the Center for Tobacco Products of the U.S. Food and Drug Administration; a commissioner for the Lancet Commission on Obesity; and a member of the Food and Nutrition Board of the National Academies of Sciences, Engineering, and Medicine. Dr. Hammond holds a Ph.D. from the University of Michigan.

**Eric Hekler, M.S., Ph.D.,** is the director of the Center for Wireless & Population Health Systems (CWPHS) in the Qualcomm Institute, an associate professor in the Department of Family Medicine & Public Health, and a faculty member of the Design Lab at the University of California, San Diego. He is a transdisciplinary researcher, educator, and practitioner in his work at the intersection of clinical health psychology, human-centered design, public health, and control systems engineering. There are three interdependent themes to his research: advancing methods for optimizing adaptive behavioral interventions; advancing methods and processes to help people help themselves; and research pipelines to achieve efficient, rigorous, context-relevant solutions for complex problems. A central guiding theme for Dr. Hekler's work is to contribute to a form of applied science that facilitates equitable participation, contribution, and benefit, with technology being used when appropriate to support this broader effort. He has authored more than 120 publications that span the many disciplines to which he contributes, with a wide range of federal and foundation funding. He is recognized internationally as an expert in the area of digital health. Dr. Hekler holds an M.S. and a Ph.D. in clinical psychology from Rutgers University.

**Erin Hennessy, M.S., M.P.H., Ph.D.,** is an assistant professor at the Friedman School of Nutrition Science and Policy in the Division of Nutrition Communications and Behavior Change at Tufts University. Through her research, she works with the ChildObesity180 initiative to advance the mission and impact of scaling evidence-based obesity prevention strategies nationwide. She is committed to working with diverse communities to promote health through better nutrition and physical activity and to training the next generation of leaders and engaged citizens. She leads an active research portfolio that includes a study to test and evaluate the use of telehealth innovations in the delivery of the Special Supplemental Nutrition Program for Women, Infants, and Children of the U.S. Department of Agriculture and co-leads a study for the National Institutes of Health, in partnership with the New York Road Runners organization, to create and implement a multilevel intervention to support physical literacy at school and at home. Her research has a strong foundation in developing innovative dietary assessment techniques, using qualitative, participatory methods and integrating novel approaches, such as agent-based modeling and social network analysis, to advance community obesity prevention interventions. Dr. Hennessy holds a B.S. in biology and a certificate in community health, an M.S. in nutrition communication from the Friedman School, an M.P.H. from the School of Medicine, and a Ph.D. in food policy and applied nutrition, all from Tufts University.

**John Jakicic, M.S., Ph.D.,** is the director of the Healthy Lifestyle Institute and the chair of the Department of Health and Physical Activity at the University of Pittsburgh. Considered a leading authority on the benefits of physical activity for weight management, he has authored more than 230 peer-reviewed publications and given more than 200 invited presentations. Dr. Jakicic has been an American College of Sports Medicine (ACSM) member for more than 30 years, serving on the ACSM board of trustees, multiple committees, and as associate editor for *Medicine & Science in Sports & Exercise.* He has also served on the board of directors for the Mid-Atlantic Chapter of ACSM. Dr. Jakicic holds an M.S. in exercise science from Slippery Rock University and a Ph.D. in exercise physiology from the University of Pittsburgh.

**Matt Kasman, M.A., Ph.D.,** is the assistant research director at the Brookings Institution Center on Social Dynamics and Policy. He has extensive experience applying systems science approaches to study the impact of public health and educational policy and practice. Dr. Kasman's recent research has focused on whole-of-community childhood obesity prevention interventions, retail tobacco control, racial disparities in exposure to HIV, access to physical activity, maternal and childhood consumption of sugar-sweetened beverages, food preference formation, college affirmative action, subsidized college tuition, school choice and student assignment algorithms, and financial literacy. Previously, he worked for software start-ups that were sold to Microsoft, Google, and Blackbaud. He is currently a fellow with the Lancet Commission on Obesity and an instructor at the Washington University Systems Science for Social Impact Summer Training Institute. Dr. Kasman holds an undergraduate degree in computer science from Boston University, an M.A. in politics and education from Columbia University, and a Ph.D. in educational policy from Stanford University.

**Shiriki K. Kumanyika, M.S., M.P.H., Ph.D.,** is an emerita professor of epidemiology at the University of Pennsylvania Perelman School of Medicine and a research professor in the Department of Community Health &

Prevention at the Dornsife School of Public Health at Drexel University. Dr. Kumanyika has an interdisciplinary background that integrates epidemiology, nutrition, social work, and public health methods and perspectives. The main themes in her research concern prevention and control of obesity and other diet-related risk factors and chronic diseases, with a particular focus on reducing health burdens in Black communities. Dr. Kumanyika is the founding chair of the Council on Black Health (formerly the African American Collaborative Obesity Research Network), a national network hosted by Drexel, that seeks to develop and promote solutions that achieve healthy Black communities. She is a member of the National Academy of Medicine. She is a past president of the American Public Health Association and has served in numerous advisory roles related to public health research and policy in the United States and abroad. At the National Academies of Sciences, Engineering, and Medicine, she chaired the Standing Committee on Obesity from 2009 until its retirement in 2013, and she currently chairs the Food and Nutrition Board. Dr. Kumanyika holds an M.S. in social work from Columbia University, an M.P.H. from Johns Hopkins University, and a Ph.D. in human nutrition from Cornell University.

**Douglas Luke, Ph.D.**, is a professor and director of the Ph.D. program in public health sciences at Washington University in St. Louis. He is a leading researcher in the areas of public health policy, systems science, and tobacco control, focusing primarily on the evaluation, dissemination, and implementation of evidence-based public health policies. Dr. Luke uses systems science methods, especially social network analysis and agent-based modeling, to address important public health problems. He has published widely on network analysis and systems science methods in public health and has written books on multilevel modeling and network analysis. Under Dr. Luke's leadership, the Center for Public Health Systems Science has used network analysis to study the diffusion of scientific innovations, to model the formation of organizational collaborations, and to study the relationship of mentoring to future scientific collaboration. In addition to his appointment at the Brown School, Dr. Luke is a member of the Institute for Public Health, the director of evaluation for the Institute of Clinical and Translational Science, and a founding member of the Washington University Network of Dissemination and Implementation Researchers. He served on an Institute of Medicine panel that produced a national report on the use of agent-based modeling for tobacco regulatory science. Dr. Luke holds a Ph.D. from the University of Illinois.

**Tiffany M. Powell-Wiley, M.P.H., M.D.**, is an Earl Stadtman tenure-track investigator at the National Institutes of Health, with joint appointments in the Cardiovascular Branch of the Division of Intramural Research at the National Heart, Lung, and Blood Institute and the Intramural Research Program of the National Institute on Minority Health and Health Disparities. She is also the chief of the Social Determinants of Obesity and Cardiovascular Risk Laboratory, which is currently focused on three main research goals for improving cardiometabolic health in high-risk communities in Washington, DC, to delineate mechanisms by which neighborhood environment influences the development of obesity, diabetes, and other markers of cardiometabolic risk; identify methods for incorporating mobile health technology to address behaviors associated with poor cardiometabolic health in resource-limited environments; and identify and characterize physiologic pathways influenced by the chronic stress that comes from living in adverse neighborhood conditions. The ultimate goal is to elucidate the pathways linked to cardiometabolic risk phenotypes and most responsive to targeted health behavior interventions. This research program is designed to leverage community-based participatory research principles, epidemiologic methods, and translational approaches to harness emerging technologies in improving the cardiometabolic health of at-risk, underserved communities most affected by health disparities. Dr. Powell-Wiley holds an M.P.H. with a concentration in epidemiology from the University of North Carolina at Chapel Hill and an M.D. from the Duke University School of Medicine.

**Nicolaas (Nico) P. Pronk, Ph.D.,** is the president of the HealthPartners Institute and the chief science officer at HealthPartners, Inc. He also holds a faculty appointment as an adjunct professor of social and behavioral sciences at the Harvard T.H. Chan School of Public Health. The HealthPartners Institute, one of the largest medical research and education centers in the Midwest, annually has about 450 studies under way; trains more than 500 medical residents and fellows and more than 500 students; and provides continuing medical education for 25,000 clinicians, as well as patient education and clinical quality improvement. HealthPartners, Inc., founded in 1957 as a cooperative, is an integrated, nonprofit, member-governed health system providing health care services and health plan financing and administration. It is the largest consumer-governed nonprofit health care organization in the United States. Dr. Pronk's work is focused on connecting evidence of effectiveness with the practical application of programs and practices, policies, and systems that measurably improve population health and well-being. His work applies to workplaces, care delivery settings, and communities and involves the development of new models for improving health and well-being at the research, practice, and policy levels. His research interests include workplace health and safety, obesity, physical activity, and systems approaches to population health and well-being. Dr. Pronk currently serves as co-chair of the U.S. Secretary of Health and

Human Services' Advisory Committee on National Health Promotion and Disease Prevention Objectives for 2030 (Healthy People 2030) and is a former member of the Community Preventive Services Task Force. He was the founding president of the International Association for Worksite Health Promotion and has served on boards and committees at the National Academies of Sciences, Engineering, and Medicine; the American Heart Association; and the Health Enhancement Research Organization, among others. He is widely published in both the scientific and practice literatures and is an international speaker on population health and health promotion. Dr. Pronk holds a Ph.D. in exercise physiology from Texas A&M University and completed postdoctoral studies in behavioral medicine at the University of Pittsburgh Medical Center at the Western Psychiatric Institute and Clinic.

**Daniel E. Rivera, M.S., Ph.D.,** is a professor of chemical engineering in the School for Engineering of Matter, Transport, and Energy and the program director of the Control Systems Engineering Laboratory at Arizona State University (ASU). Prior to joining ASU, he was an associate research engineer in the Control Systems Section of Shell Development Company. He has been a visiting researcher with the Division of Automatic Control at Linköping University, Sweden; the Honeywell Technology Center; the Saints Cyril and Methodius University in Skopje, Macedonia; the National Distance Learning University in Madrid, Spain; and the University of Almería in Andalucía, Spain. Dr. Rivera's research interests include robust process control; system identification; and the application of control engineering principles to problems in process systems, supply chain management, and prevention and treatment interventions in behavioral medicine. He was chosen as the 1994–1995 outstanding undergraduate educator by the ASU student chapter of the American Institute of Chemical Engineers and was the recipient of a Teaching Excellence Award from ASU's College of Engineering and Applied Sciences. He has also received a Mentored Quantitative Research Career Development Award from the National Institutes of Health to study control systems approaches for fighting drug abuse. Dr. Rivera holds a B.S. from the University of Rochester, an M.S. from the University of Wisconsin–Madison, and a Ph.D. in chemical engineering from the California Institute of Technology.

**Bonnie Spring, Ph.D.,** is a professor of preventive medicine, psychology, psychiatry, and public health at Northwestern University and the director of its Center for Behavior and Health in the Institute for Public Health and Medicine. She is also the team science director for the Northwestern University Clinical and Translational Sciences Institute and the program co-leader for cancer prevention at the Robert Lurie Comprehensive Cancer Center. She studies technology-supported interventions to promote healthy change in multiple chronic disease risk behaviors, particularly a poor-quality diet, overeating, physical inactivity, and smoking. Her current work involves the use of wearable sensors to predict and preempt relapse to smoking, optimize treatment for obesity, and prevent loss of cardiovascular health among college students. A past president of the Society for Behavioral Medicine (SBM), she is a recipient of SBM's awards for distinguished research mentor, research to practice translation, outstanding optimization research, and distinguished leadership, as well as the founding editor of its journal, *Translational Behavioral Medicine: Practice, Policy, Research*. Dr. Spring is also a recipient of the Obesity Society's e-Health Pioneer Award and past chair of the American Heart Association's Behavior Change Committee. She recently chaired the Psychosocial Risk and Disease Prevention standing study section of the National Institutes of Health (NIH). A past chair of the Board of Scientific Affairs of the American Psychological Association (APA), she also received an APA presidential citation for innovative research and leadership in health psychology and vision in incorporating technology into practice and training. Her NIH-supported science of team science and evidence-based practice open-access learning modules have been used by more than 50,000 learners worldwide. Dr. Spring holds a Ph.D. from Harvard University.